THE KETO CHAFFLE COOK

Easy Low-Carb Recipes To Lose Weight

CONTENTS

Oreo Keto Chaffles

Gingerbread Chaffle

Chocolate Peanut Butter Chaffle

Pumpkin Pecan Chaffles

Italian Cream Chaffle Sandwich-Cake

Chocolate Cherry Chaffles

Banana Nut Chaffle

Savory Chaffles

Belgium Chaffles

Bacon Chaffles

Crispy Bagel Chaffles

Bacon And Ham Chaffle Sandwich

Parmesan Garlic Chaffle

Buffalo Chicken Chaffles

Garlic Cheese Chaffle Bread Sticks

Chaffle Bruschetta

Pizza Chaffle

Eggs Benedict Chaffle

Zucchini Chaffle

Breakfast Chaffle

Cheddar Jalapeño Chaffle

Broccoli and Cheese Chaffles

Hash Brown Chaffle

Chicken Parmesan Chaffle

Taco Chaffle Shell

Pulled Pork Chaffle

Chicken Bacon Chaffle

Chaffle Cuban Sandwich

Salmon Chaffles

Chaffle Katsu Sandwich

Cauliflower Chaffle

Vegan Chaffle

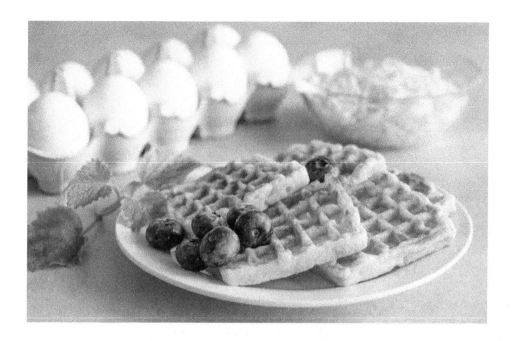

INTRODUCTION

W affles are amazing. There are so many types of waffles, it's easy to find one to love. Or even make a brand new flavor. Take a classic waffle, put something unique on top, or change a batter a little bit, and voila, you have invented a new waffle!

But what if you happen to be on a keto diet? How can you still enjoy waffles? The answer is the chaffle!

Chaffles are amazing on their own, with a unique, distinct taste. Like regular waffles, there are enough types for anyone to find a favorite.

The purpose of this book is to introduce the reader into the chaffle making process. To be a guide to everything related to this process. And I hope, it will do just that.

So, flip this page and get started! Chaffles are waiting to be baked and enjoyed!

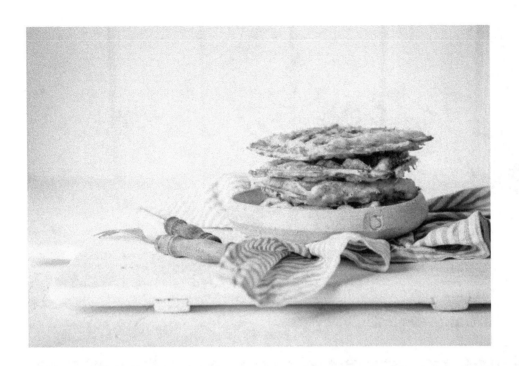

CHAPTER 1. WHAT IS KETO AND WHY IS IT GOOD FOR YOU?

KETO DIET EXPLAINED

Keto diet is short for "ketogenic." This is a high-fat content diet that's purpose is turning your body into a true fat-burning machine.

The way keto diet achieves that is by changing the way your body converts food into energy. Usually, your body takes energy from carbohydrates by turning them in glucose. When you eat very few carbs and a lot of fat, it puts you in ketosis. Glucose is to carbohydrates ketones are to fat.

And what is Ketosis?

The term ketosis relates to a byproduct of breaking down fat into useable energy, called ketones.

This fat can be derived from fat stores of the body or directly from a diet. Ketosis is caused by diet is referred to as "nutritional ketosis." Ketones are used by the body to directly power itself.

This process of breaking down fat into useful energy is similar to the process that carbohydrates undergo when turned into glucose to fuel the body. In other words, glucose is to carbohydrates ketones are to fat.

What are ketones?

When your body doesn't get enough glucose from your diet, your liver starts to turn your body's fat and fat from your diet into molecules called ketones, an alternative source of fuel.

The keto diet is the main way to get your body running on ketones. Other ways include intermittent fasting, taking certain keto supplements, and using up your glucose reserves by exercising.

KETOGENIC HEALTH BENEFITS

Burns body fat

When you're on a keto diet, your body uses fat from your diet as well as stored body fat for energy. This helps people stay at a healthy weight.

Reduces appetite

Ketones can suppress ghrelin — your hunger hormone — and increase cholecystokinin (CCK), which makes you feel full. Reduced appetite makes it easier to go without eating for longer periods, which encourages your body to resort to its fat stores for energy.

Reduces inflammation

Inflammation is your body's natural reaction to an invader it considers harmful. But too much inflammation raises your risk of health and digestion problems. A keto diet is able to reduce inflammation in the body by switching off the inflammatory mechanisms and producing fewer free radicals.

Fuels your brain

Ketones can provide a good portion of your brain's energy needs, more than the energy you get from glucose. The brain is made up of more than 60% fat.

That means it highly needs fat to work as it should, and the quality fats you eat on a ketogenic diet are ideal for feeding the brain.

Increases energy

When your body uses ketones for fuel, the same energy slumps as when you're eating a lot of carbs don't happen. Your body can easily tap into its fat stores for energy when your metabolism is in fat-burning mode. That means no more energy slumps or brain fog. Ketosis also helps to create more mitochondria, the power generators in your cells. Having more energy in your cells results in more energy to get stuff done.

Curbs cravings

Fat is a satiating macronutrient. You eat more smart fats on keto, you feel fuller, longer.

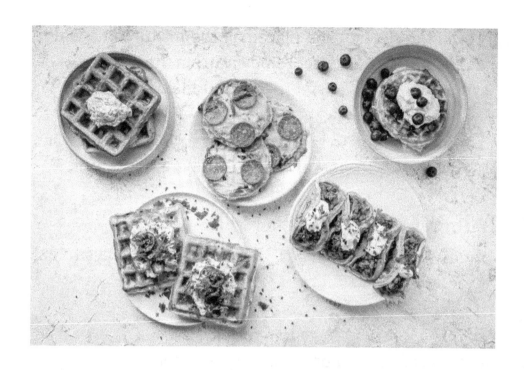

CHAPTER 2. WHAT IS A KETO CHAFFLE?

WAFFLES VS. CHAFFLES

A chaffle is a keto waffle. It's called a chaffle because one of its primary ingredients is shredded cheese, hence the CHaffle instead of Waffle because chaffles are cheese waffles. Pretty cool, right?

Waffles are usually made of a flour-based batter, but a chaffle is made of eggs and cheese. It sounds odd, but it actually works!

Chaffles are a great way for those on the keto diet to get their waffle fix. They're also a great way to eat fewer carbs while still eating what you want! Even if it is a modified version. There are also endless chaffle ingredient combinations.

HOW A BASIC CHAFFLE IS MADE

A basic chaffle is made of just two ingredients: ½ cup of shredded cheese, like mozzarella, and 1 large egg.

Finely shredded cheese or thicker shreds work, it's completely up to you.

You whisk the egg, stir in the cheese, and place half the mixture in a waffle maker at a time for 2-3 minutes. Then, after removing from the waffle maker, let them sit for 1-2 minutes. They'll crisp up like a normal waffle would as they set.

You can add almond or coconut flour to give it a more bread-like texture. One teaspoon of either is a good place to start and adjust to your preferences.

HOW TO EAT/SERVE A BASIC CHAFFLE

Even though they are as simple as it can get, there are a lot of ways to eat chaffles:

Plain

Chaffles are great as a breakfast food on their own. You can serve them up alongside bacon, avocado, eggs, and other standard keto breakfast foods.

Keto chaffle sandwich

You can make two chaffles and use them to replace the bread for your favorite sandwich. Chaffles are great as the bread for breakfast sandwiches, turkey clubs, or any other keto-friendly sandwiches.

Chaffle dessert

You can try a sweet chaffle variation and serve it with your favorite keto ice cream or keto maple syrup.

You can also customize your chaffle in all kinds of ways:

Different cheeses

Mozzarella, Cheddar, Parmesan, Colby Jack, Philadelphia cream cheese — any cheese that melts well will work with a chaffle. Different cheeses produce slightly different textures and different flavors.

Sweeteners

You can add your favorite keto sweetener, like stevia or sucralose, to the batter before you fry it up. You can also try adding chocolate chips or lowsugar fruits like strawberries or blueberries.

Herbs and spices

Add savory ingredients like herbs and spices to your chaffle. For a pizza chaffle, add oregano, garlic powder, and diced pepperoni to the batter, with tomato sauce and extra cheese on top. Or you could use cream cheese and add everything bagel seasoning to the batter for an everything bagel chaffle. Serve with more cream cheese on top, capers, onions, and smoked salmon.

Give chaffles a try and come up with your own favorite variations. They're an excellent addition to a ketogenic diet and a lot of fun to experiment with within the kitchen. And for inspiration and more awesome keto food, check out all our low-carb recipes.

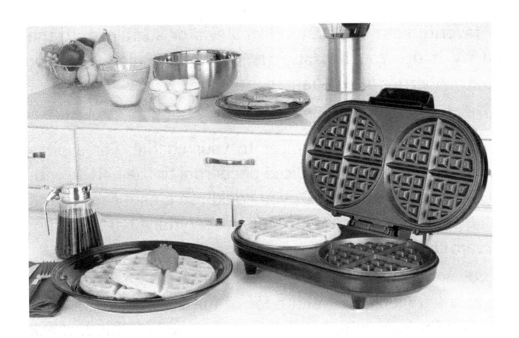

CHAPTER 3. CHAFFLE MACHINES AND TIPS

DIFFERENT CHAFFLE MAKERS, HOW TO CHOOSE

A chaffle maker and a waffle maker is actually the same thing. It is a simple appliance that allows you to create amazing treats, and there is a wide range of different models and products intended to bring you the fluffiest chaffles and waffles possible.

You might not think of it, but the world of waffle-chaffle makers can be quite vast with a number of different types to choose from. Because there are that many different types of chaffles and waffles, the devices used to create them also have to be different.

Here are the most popular types and what they offer as a chaffle/waffle maker:

Classic round waffle makers

They have a characteristic round shape, and they produce waffles that are thinner than Belgian waffle makers. Many people prefer non-Belgian waffle makers as they resemble the thinner ready-made varieties found in stores.

Square waffle makers

The square shape is the most popular along with the circle. Outcome waffles are usually cut into four smaller pieces. Belgian waffles are also this shape. However, the difference is in thickness.

Belgian waffle makers

Arguably, the most popular type of machine as a whole. The Belgian waffle makers cook square waffles, which can be pretty thick. A Belgian waffle vs. regular waffle ordinarily ranges up from 1" to 1½" in thickness, and they have a fluffy inside and a crispy outside.

Ceramic waffle makers

These are great alternatives to Teflon coated waffle makers, and many people believe the ceramic waffle maker is easier to clean and that they influence the flavor of the waffle less than metal waffle makers. Another benefit is that ceramic is almost free from harmful chemicals if compared to normal kitchenware.

Waffle irons

Technically speaking, a waffle iron is commonly referred to as a stovetop waffle maker because it makes waffles over the stove. However, many people still use the term interchangeably with electric waffle makers.

Flip waffle makers

A waffle flip is a device that is made to allow flipping the batter around once it is poured in. It is designed for even cooking the batter over the grill. Some people like this style better than the traditional waffle press as it ensures that there's no uncooked batter in the finished product, and makes less mess.

So, there are tons of special features, variations, and other things you need to consider before making your purchase. And this is indeed great because it lets you find the one to suit your exact needs.

Here are just some of the separate things that are worth considering:

Output

Output refers to how many waffles at a time the machine can make, and your choice should depend on how many people you have to feed and their appetite. Most standard machines produce just one or two waffles. However, some of them can make up to eight waffles and even beyond in commercialstyle waffle makers.

Waffle style

Waffles come in many different styles, from classic Belgian waffles to traditional American waffles, so you have many specific styles of waffle makers to choose from.

Shape

Fancy waffle maker's shapes were a bestseller in recent years. The ability to transform your favorite treat into a star or heart was such a hit! These come either as an insert to your waffle maker, or a separate machine. But the most common shape nowadays still remains the classic square or a circle.

Thickness

You can pick a waffle maker depending on how thick you like your waffles. Most waffles range from thin, of around ½ inch, to thick, of around 1½ inch.

Grill surface

Look for a non-stick grill surface, preferably something coated with Teflon, or just made from ceramic. This will help in two ways: your waffles won't stick when you try to get them, and, consequently, the cleanup will be considerably easier.

Lights and display

Most modern machines have at least a small light indicator that shows when the waffle maker is heated up and ready to cook the batter. More advanced models might also feature another light to show when your waffle is approximately done and even a digital display for further information.

Digital timer

If you don't use a timer in waffle making, you are more prone to end up under or overcooking your waffle. Both are usually to hard to enjoy, but undercooked waffles additionally stick in the griddle, becoming a mess to dig out! To prevent all of this, some waffle makers have convenient built-in countdown timers.

Flip ability

Traditionally, flip waffle makers were usually qualified as professional only, which was making them quite expensive. However, nowadays, there are many new affordable designs with a flip function. They help to achieve an even spread of batter on the grill.

There are many smaller features that might attract some users, such as browning settings and drip trays. However, they are all optional and not necessary.

Thankfully, the range of today's waffle makers is more diverse and accessible than ever before! The choices are all quite enticing. Shop smart and think about what you really want from your waffle maker before pulling the trigger.

CHAFFLE MAKING TIPS, FREQUENTLY ASKED QUESTIONS

CAN YOU TASTE THE CHEESE IN A SWEET KETO CHAFFLE?

Of course, this question is subjective as one person's taste buds are different from others, but it partly depends on how distinct the taste of the cheese that was used is.

WHAT DO YOU MEAN BY SAVORY?

Unlike chaffles served with sugar-free syrup or fresh berries, savory chaffles aren't sweet. Instead, they taste more like a traditional bread and can be used to make personal pan pizzas, crispy keto taco shells, and more.

VARIETIES OF CHEESE FOR CHAFFLES:

There are many different kinds of cheese that you can use in keto chaffle recipes. The most suitable are listed below. You can also mix different cheeses together.

So:

- ☐ Colby Jack
- ☐ Monterey Jack
- ☐ White Cheddar Cheese
- ☐ Mild Cheddar & Sharp Cheddar
- ☐ Parmesan Cheese ☐ Mozzarella

You can use cream cheese like Philadelphia in place of cheese, but the texture will be different. Cream cheese makes much softer, unstructured chaffles.

ALMOND/COCONUT FLOUR IN CHAFFLES:

Why do some recipes require adding flour, and some don't?

Coconut flour gives chaffles a bit of a bread-like texture, especially in sweet chaffle recipes. Usually, just 1 tsp of coconut flour along with ¼ tsp of baking powder is enough.

If using almond flour instead, you should make an amount conversion. The standard conversion in keto recipes is one part coconut flour to four parts almond flour, but that isn't the case with chaffles. Since you only use a small amount of coconut flour in recipes, the overall conversion rate is just one teaspoon coconut flour equals one tablespoon almond flour.

Why do some recipes require adding flour, and some don't?

While both adding and not adding flour to the same recipe may result okay, sometimes a bit of coconut or almond flour garners a better overall taste, especially in sweet recipes.

WHAT IS THE PURPOSE OF BAKING POWDER?

The baking powder adds bubbles to the chaffle batter, causing them to puff up a bit and be less dense.

HOW DO I STORE CHAFFLES?

Any plastic container that you find okay to use in the freezer will do. Even freezer bags. If they are basic chaffles, let them cool before setting them in the freezer. The heat and condensation will make them stick. Other chaffles covered in crazy ingredients, however, you may want to separate them with parchment paper or something similar.

HOW DO I REHEAT CHAFFLES?

You can reheat chaffles in several different ways, such as in the oven, toaster, air fryer, or skillet. You can also put them back into the waffle maker to heat up and make them crispy again.

Just don't use a microwave, they don't taste fresh after that.

HOW DO I CLEAN MY WAFFLE MAKER?

There is a lot of ways. One of them is putting a wet cloth in and letting the steam loosen everything up after unplugging it. Then, when it's cool, use it to wipe it off. The heat will kill everything on it. There are also all sorts of dishwashing gadgets out there that can get between the grooves if needed.

WHY DOES THE CHAFFLE STICK?

There are a few reasons why it may happen:

☐ Your waffle maker's surface may be wearing out from general use.

☐ You may not be letting the batter to cook long enough. ☐
The type of chaffle you're cooking is just a bit stickier.

CHAPTER 4. RECIPES

SWEET CHAFFLES

BASIC KETO CHAFFLES

SERVINGS: 2 PREP TIME: 5 min. COOK TIME: 5 min.

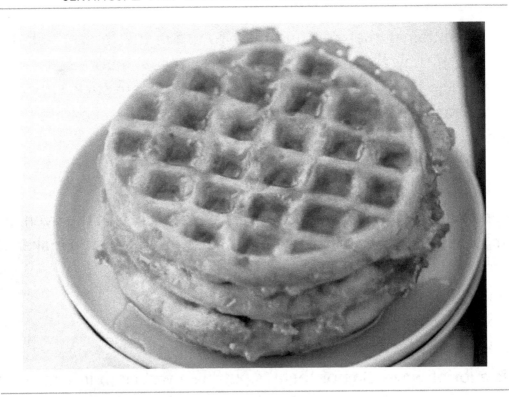

CARBS – 1 g FAT – 12 g PROTEIN – 9 g CALORIES – 150

Ingredients

- *1 egg*

½ cup shredded Cheddar cheese

Directions

1. Turn on waffle maker to heat and oil it with cooking spray.
2. Whisk egg in a bowl until well beaten.
3. Add cheese to the egg and stir well to combine.
4. Pour ½ batter into the waffle maker and close the top. Cook for 3-5 minutes.
5. Transfer chaffle to a plate and set aside for 2-3 minutes to crisp up.
6. Repeat for remaining batter.

BLUEBERRY CINNAMON CHAFFLES

SERVINGS: 3 PREP TIME: 5 min. COOK TIME: 10 min.

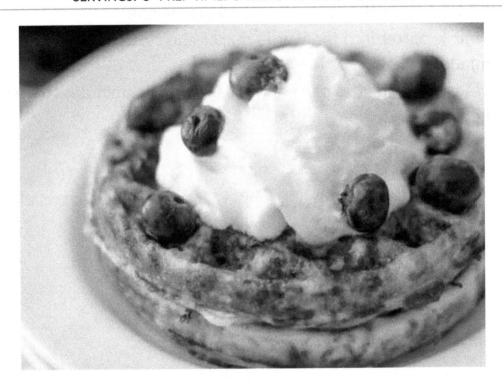

CARBS – 9 g FAT – 12 g PROTEIN – 13 g CALORIES – 193

Ingredients

- *1 cup shredded mozzarella cheese*
- *3 Tbsp almond flour*
- *2 eggs*
- *2 tsp Swerve or granulated sweetener of choice*
- *1 tsp cinnamon*

½ tsp baking powder
½ cup fresh blueberries
½ tsp of powdered Swerve

Directions

1. Turn on waffle maker to heat and oil it with cooking spray.
2. Mix eggs, flour, mozzarella, cinnamon, vanilla extract, sweetener, and baking powder in a bowl until well combined.
3. Add in blueberries.
4. Pour ¼ batter into each waffle mold.
5. Close and cook for 8 minutes.
6. If it's crispy and the waffle maker opens without pulling the chaffles apart, the chaffle is ready. If not, close and cook for 1-2 minutes more.

7. Serve with favorite topping and more blueberries.

CINNAMON ROLL CHAFFLES

SERVINGS: 3 PREP TIME: 15 min. COOK TIME: 25 min.

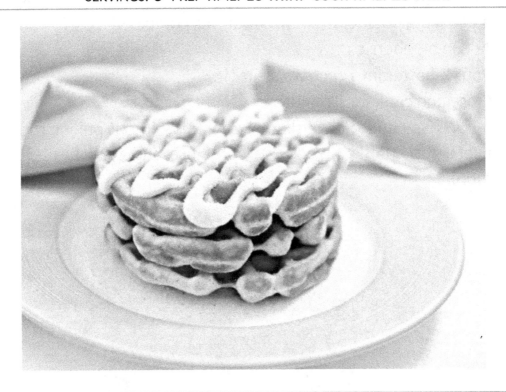

CARBS – 31 g FAT – 15 g PROTEIN – 9 g CALORIES – 195

Ingredients

FOR THE BATTER:

- ½ cup shredded mozzarella cheese
- 2 Tbsp golden monk fruit sweetener
- 2 Tbsp SunButter

1 egg

1 Tbsp coconut flour

2 tsp cinnamon

¼ tsp vanilla extract

⅛ tsp baking powder

FOR THE FROSTING:

- *¼ cup powdered monk fruit sweetener*
- *1 Tbsp cream cheese*
- *¾ Tbsp butter, melted*
- *¼ tsp vanilla extract*
- *1 Tbsp unsweetened coconut milk*

FOR THE COATING:

- *1 tsp cinnamon*
- *1 tsp golden monk fruit sweetener*

Directions

1. Turn on waffle maker to heat and oil it with cooking spray.
2. Combine all batter components in a bowl, then set aside and leave for 3-5 minutes.
3. In another bowl, whisk all frosting components until well-combined.
4. Divide batter into 3 portions and spoon 1 part into the waffle maker.
5. Cook for 2-4 minutes, until golden brown.
6. Open and let chaffle cool for 30 seconds in waffle maker before you transfer it to a plate.
7. Repeat with remaining batter.
8. While chaffles are warm, sprinkle with cinnamon and sweetener coating. When cooled a little, drizzle with icing.

YOGURT CHAFFLES

SERVINGS: 3 PREP TIME: 5 min. + overnight COOK TIME: 10 min.

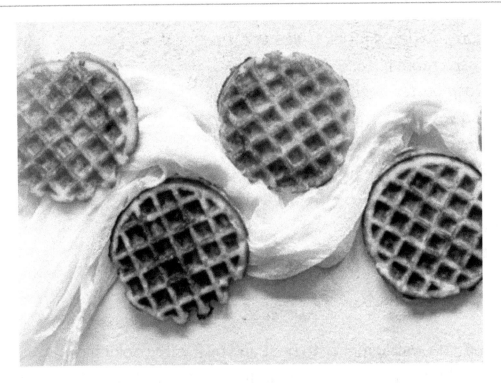

CARBS – 2 g FAT – 5 g PROTEIN – 4 g CALORIES – 93

Ingredients

- ½ cup shredded mozzarella
- 1 egg
- 2 Tbsp ground almonds
- ½ tsp psyllium husk
- ¼ tsp baking powder

1 Tbsp yogurt

Directions

1. Turn on waffle maker to heat and oil it with cooking spray.
2. Whisk eggs in a bowl.
3. Add in remaining ingredients except mozzarella and mix well.
4. Add mozzarella and mix once again. Let it sit for 5 minutes.
5. Add ⅓ cup batter into each waffle mold.
6. Close and cook for 4-5 minutes.

7. Repeat with remaining batter.

CHOCOLATE CHAFFLES

SERVINGS: 2 PREP TIME: 1 min. COOK TIME: 10 min.

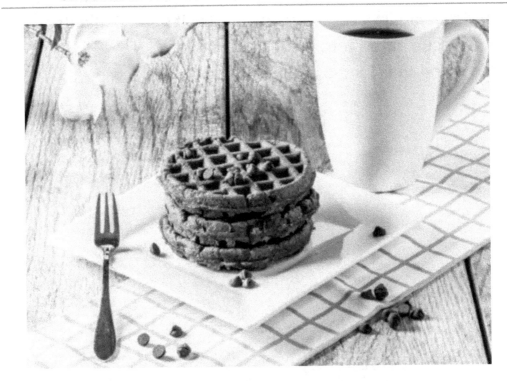

CARBS – 6 g FAT – 24 g PROTEIN – 15 g CALORIES – 296

Ingredients

- ¾ cup shredded mozzarella
- 1 large egg
- 2 Tbsp almond flour
- 2 Tbsp allulose

½ Tbsp melted butter
1½ Tbsp cocoa powder
½ tsp vanilla extract
½ tsp psyllium husk powder
¼ tsp baking powder

Directions

1. Turn on waffle maker to heat and oil it with cooking spray.
2. Mix all ingredients in a small bowl.
3. Pour ¼ cup batter into a 4-inch waffle maker.
4. Cook for 2-3 minutes, or until crispy.
5. Transfer chaffle to a plate and set aside.

6. Repeat with remaining batter.

RASPBERRY CHAFFLES

SERVINGS: 2 PREP TIME: 5 min. COOK TIME: 5 min.

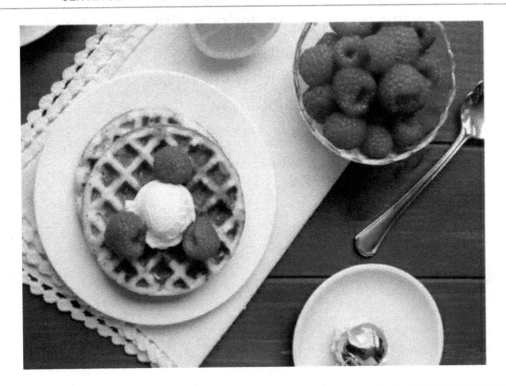

CARBS – 5 g FAT – 11 g PROTEIN – 24 g CALORIES – 300

Ingredients

- *4 Tbsp almond flour*
- *4 large eggs*
- *2 ⅓ cup shredded mozzarella cheese*
- *1 tsp vanilla extract*

1 Tbsp erythritol sweetener
1½ tsp baking powder
½ cup raspberries

Directions

1. Turn on waffle maker to heat and oil it with cooking spray.
2. Mix almond flour, sweetener, and baking powder in a bowl.
3. Add cheese, eggs, and vanilla extract, and mix until well-combined.
4. Add 1 portion of batter to waffle maker and spread it evenly. Close and cook for 3-4 minutes, or until golden.
5. Repeat until remaining batter is used.

6. Serve with raspberries.

CINNAMON CHAFFLE

SERVINGS: 1 PREP TIME: 5 min. COOK TIME: 5 min.

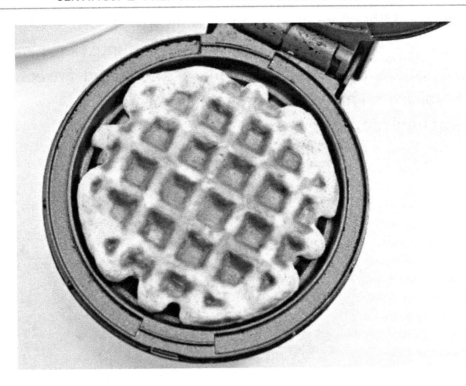

CARBS – 1 g FAT – 8 g PROTEIN – 9 g CALORIES – 120

Ingredients

- *1 egg*
- *1 cup shredded mozzarella cheese*
- *½ tsp vanilla*
- *½ tsp cinnamon*

Directions

1. Turn on waffle maker to heat and oil it with cooking spray.
2. Whisk egg and mozzarella together in a bowl.
3. Stir in vanilla and cinnamon.
4. Place half of the batter into waffle maker. Cook for 2-3 minutes.
5. Repeat with remaining batter.

STRAWBERRY SHORTCAKE CHAFFLES

SERVINGS: 1 PREP TIME: 20 min. COOK TIME: 25 min.

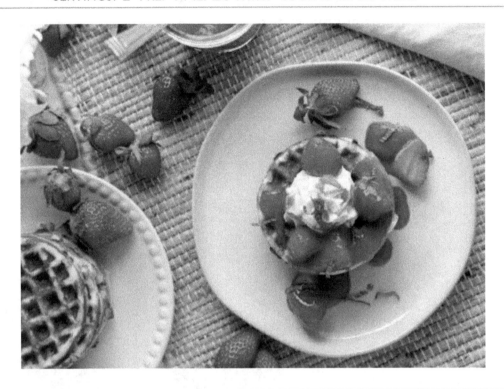

CARBS – 5 g FAT – 14 g PROTEIN – 12 g CALORIES – 218

Ingredients

FOR THE BATTER:

- 1 egg
- ¼ cup mozzarella cheese
- 1   Tbsp cream cheese¼ tsp baking
- powder
-
-

2 strawberries, sliced

1 tsp strawberry extract

FOR THE GLAZE:

- *1 Tbsp cream cheese*
- *¼ tsp strawberry extract*
- *1 Tbsp monk fruit confectioners blend*

FOR THE WHIPPED CREAM:

- *1 cup heavy whipping cream*
- *1 tsp vanilla*
- *1 Tbsp monk fruit*

Directions

1. Turn on waffle maker to heat and oil it with cooking spray.
2. Beat egg in a small bowl.
3. Add remaining batter components.
4. Divide the mixture in half.
5. Cook one half of the batter in a waffle maker for 4 minutes, or until golden brown.
6. Repeat with remaining batter
7. Mix all glaze ingredients and spread over each warm chaffle.
8. Mix all whipped cream ingredients and whip until it starts to form peaks.
9. Top each waffle with whipped cream and strawberries.

BLUEBERRY CHAFFLES

SERVINGS: 1 PREP TIME: 5 min. COOK TIME: 10 min.

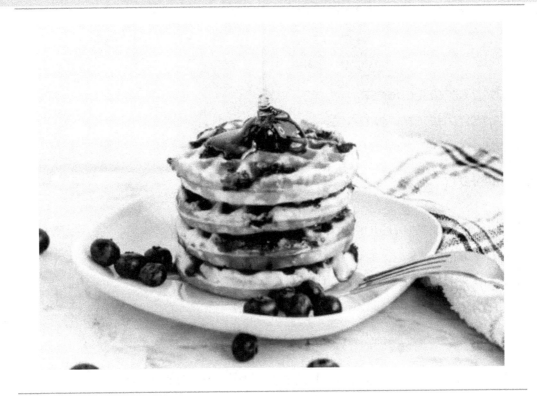

CARBS – 8 g FAT – 20 g PROTEIN – 20 g CALORIES – 296

Ingredients

- 1 egg
- ½ cup shredded mozzarella cheese
- 1 Tbsp almond flour
- 1   Tbsp swerve
- ½ tsp ground cinnamon
- ½ tsp vanilla extract
- 2   Tbsp frozen blueberries

¼ cup keto-friendly maple syrup

Directions

1. Turn on waffle maker to heat and oil it with cooking spray.
2. Mix egg, mozzarella, almond flour, cinnamon, and vanilla in a small bowl.
3. Divide mixture in half.
4. Spread one half of batter in waffle maker and top with half of berries. Cook for 5-7 minutes, until golden brown.
5. Repeat with remaining mixture.

6. Let it cool slightly, and serve with keto-friendly maple syrup.

GLAZED CHAFFLES

SERVINGS: 2 PREP TIME: 10 min. COOK TIME: 5 min.

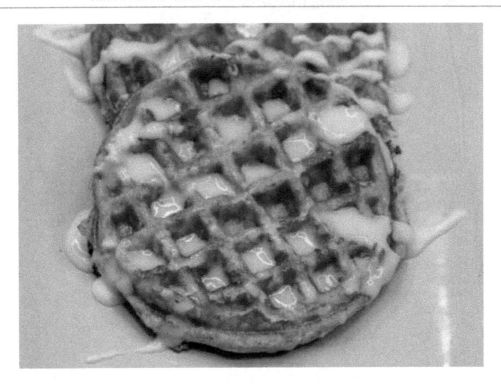

CARBS – 4 g FAT – 6 g PROTEIN – 4 g CALORIES – 130

Ingredients

- ½ cup mozzarella shredded cheese
- ⅛ cup cream cheese
- 2 Tbsp unflavored whey protein isolate
- 2 Tbsp swerve confectioners sugar substitute
- ½ tsp baking powder

½ tsp vanilla extract

1 egg

FOR THE GLAZE TOPPING:

- *2   Tbsp heavy whipping cream*
- *3-4 Tbsp swerve confectioners sugar substitute*
- *½ tsp vanilla extract*

Directions

1. Turn on waffle maker to heat and oil it with cooking spray.
2. In a microwave-safe bowl, mix mozzarella and cream cheese. Heat at 30 second intervals until melted and fully combined.
3. Add protein, 2 Tbsp sweetener, baking powder to cheese. Knead with hands until well incorporated.
4. Place dough into a mixing bowl and beat in egg and vanilla until a smooth batter forms.
5. Put ⅓ of the batter into waffle maker, and cook for 3-5 minutes, until golden brown.
6. Repeat until all 3 chaffles are made.
7. Beat glaze ingredients in a bowl and pour over chaffles before serving.

CREAM MINI-CHAFFLES

SERVINGS: 2 PREP TIME: 5 min. COOK TIME: 10 min.

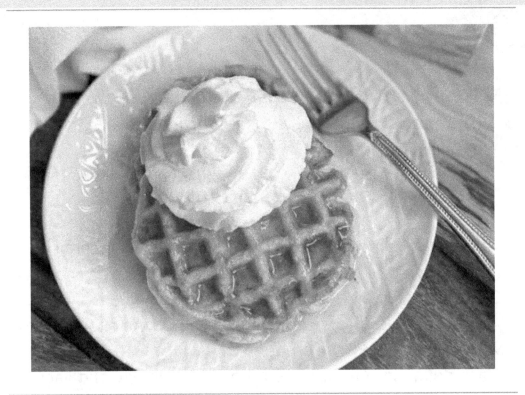

CARBS – 4 g   FAT – 6 g   PROTEIN – 2 g   CALORIES – 73

Ingredients

- 2 tsp coconut flour
- 4 tsp swerve/monk fruit
- ¼ tsp baking powder
- 1 egg
- 1 oz cream cheese
- ½ tsp vanilla extract

Directions

1. Turn on waffle maker to heat and oil it with cooking spray.

2. Mix swerve/monk fruit, coconut flour, and baking powder in a small mixing bowl.
3. Add cream cheese, egg, vanilla extract, and whisk until wellcombined.
4. Add batter into waffle maker and cook for 3-4 minutes, until golden brown.

5. Serve with your favorite toppings.

LEMON CURD CHAFFLES

SERVINGS: 1   PREP TIME: 45 min.   COOK TIME: 5 min.

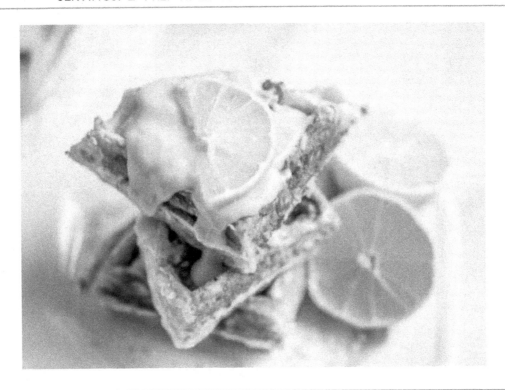

CARBS – 6 g   FAT – 24 g   PROTEIN – 15 g   CALORIES –302

Ingredients

- 3 large eggs
- 4 oz cream cheese, softened
- 1 Tbsp low carb sweetener
- 1 tsp vanilla extract
- ¾ cup mozzarella cheese, shredded

3 Tbsp coconut flour
1 tsp baking powder
⅓ tsp salt

FOR THE LEMON CURD:

- *½-1 cup water*
- *5 egg yolks*
- *½ cup lemon juice*
- *½ cup powdered sweetener*
- *2 Tbsp fresh lemon zest*
- *1 tsp vanilla extract*
- *Pinch of salt*

8 Tbsp cold butter, cubed

Directions

1. Pour water into a saucepan and heat over medium until it reaches a soft boil. Start with ½ cup and add more if needed.
2. Whisk yolks, lemon juice, lemon zest, powdered sweetener, vanilla, and salt in a medium heat-proof bowl. Leave to set for 5-6 minutes.
3. Place bowl onto saucepan and heat. The bowl shouldn't be touching water.
4. Whisk mixture for 8-10 minutes, or until it begins to thicken.
5. Add butter cubes and whisk for 5-7 minutes, until it thickens.
6. When it lightly coats the back of a spoon, remove from heat.
7. Refrigerate until cool, allowing it to continue thickening.
8. Turn on waffle maker to heat and oil it with cooking spray.
9. Add baking powder, coconut flour, and salt in a small bowl. Mix well and set aside.
10. Add eggs, cream cheese, sweetener, and vanilla in a separate bowl. Using a hand beater, beat until frothy.
11. Add mozzarella to egg mixture and beat again.

12. Add dry ingredients and mix until well-combined.
13. Add batter to waffle maker and cook for 3-4 minutes.
14. Transfer to a plate and top with lemon curd before serving.

CHOCOLATE VANILLA CHAFFLES

SERVINGS: 2 PREP TIME: 5 min. COOK TIME: 5 min.

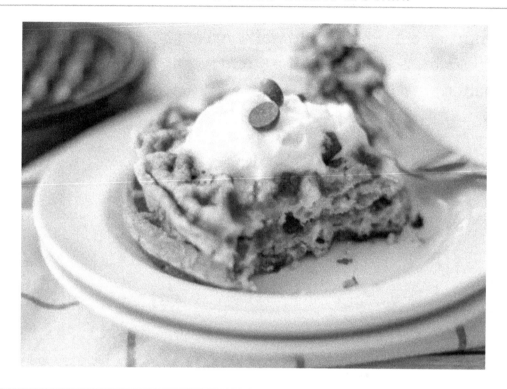

CARBS – 23 g FAT – 3 g PROTEIN – 4 g CALORIES – 134

Ingredients

- ½ cup shredded mozzarella cheese
- 1 egg
- 1 Tbsp granulated sweetener
- 1 tsp vanilla extract
- 1 Tbsp sugar-free chocolate chips
- 2 Tbsp almond meal/flour

Directions

1. Turn on waffle maker to heat and oil it with cooking spray.
2. Mix all components in a bowl until combined.
3. Pour half of the batter into waffle maker.
4. Cook for 2-4 minutes, then remove and repeat with remaining batter.

5. Top with more chips and favorite toppings.

CHAFFLE CHURROS

SERVINGS: 2 PREP TIME: 10 min. COOK TIME: 5 min.

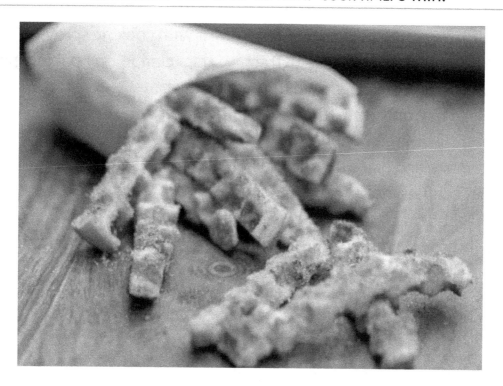

CARBS – 5 g FAT – 6 g PROTEIN – 5 g CALORIES – 76

Ingredients

- *1 egg*
- *1 Tbsp almond flour*
- *½ tsp vanilla extract*
- *1 tsp cinnamon, divided*
- *¼ tsp baking powder*
- *½ cup shredded mozzarella*

1 Tbsp swerve confectioners sugar substitute

1 Tbsp swerve brown sugar substitute

1 Tbsp butter, melted

Directions

1. Turn on waffle maker to heat and oil it with cooking spray.
2. Mix egg, flour, vanilla extract, ½ tsp cinnamon, baking powder, mozzarella, and sugar substitute in a bowl.
3. Place half of the mixture into waffle maker and cook for 3-5 minutes, or until desired doneness.
4. Remove and place the second half of the batter into the maker.
5. Cut chaffles into strips.
6. Place strips in a bowl and cover with melted butter.
7. Mix brown sugar substitute and the remaining cinnamon in a bowl.

8. Pour sugar mixture over the strips and toss to coat them well.

PEANUT BUTTER CHAFFLE

SERVINGS: 2 PREP TIME: 5 min. COOK TIME: 5 min.

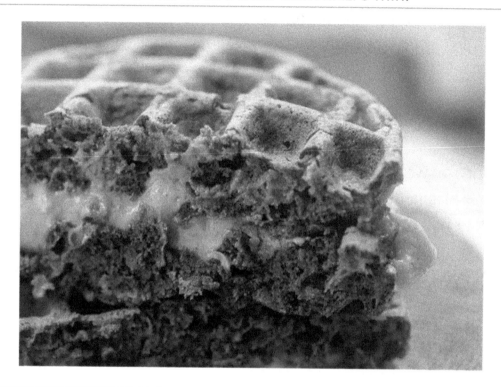

CARBS – 7 g FAT – 21 g PROTEIN – 9 g CALORIES – 264

Ingredients

- 1 egg
- 1 Tbsp heavy cream
- 1 Tbsp unsweetened cocoa
- 1 Tbsp lakanto powdered sweetener
- 1 tsp coconut flour
- ½ tsp vanilla extract
-

½ tsp cake batter flavor

¼ tsp baking powder

FOR THE FILLING:

- 3 Tbsp all-natural peanut butter
- 2 tsp lakanto powdered sweetener
- 2 Tbsp heavy cream

Directions

1. Turn on waffle maker to heat and oil it with cooking spray.
2. Mix all chaffle components in a small bowl.
3. Pour half of the mixture into waffle maker. Cook for 3-5 minutes.
4. Remove and repeat for remaining batter.
5. Allow chaffles to sit for 4-5 minutes so that they crisp up.

6. Mix filling ingredients together and spread it between chaffles.

CINNAMON PECAN CHAFFLES

SERVINGS: 1 PREP TIME: 20 min. + 12 h. COOK TIME: 40 min.

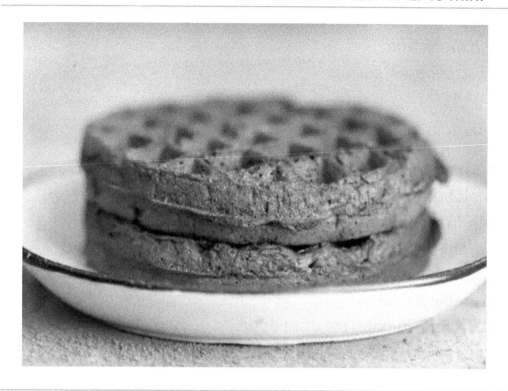

CARBS – 8 g FAT – 35 g PROTEIN – 10 g CALORIES – 391

Ingredients

- 1 Tbsp butter
- 1 egg
- ½ tsp vanilla
- 2 Tbsp almond flour
- 1 Tbsp coconut flour
- ⅛ tsp baking powder

1 Tbsp monk fruit

FOR THE CRUMBLE:

- *½ tsp cinnamon*
- *1 Tbsp melted butter*
- *1 tsp monk fruit*
- *1 Tbsp chopped pecans*

Directions

1. Turn on waffle maker to heat and oil it with cooking spray.
2. Melt butter in a bowl, then mix in the egg and vanilla.
3. Mix in remaining chaffle ingredients.
4. Combine crumble ingredients in a separate bowl.
5. Pour half of the chaffle mix into waffle maker. Top with half of crumble mixture.
6. Cook for 5 minutes, or until done.
7. Repeat with the other half of the batter.

ALMOND FLOUR CHAFFLES

SERVINGS: **2** PREP TIME: **10 min.** COOK TIME: **20 min.**

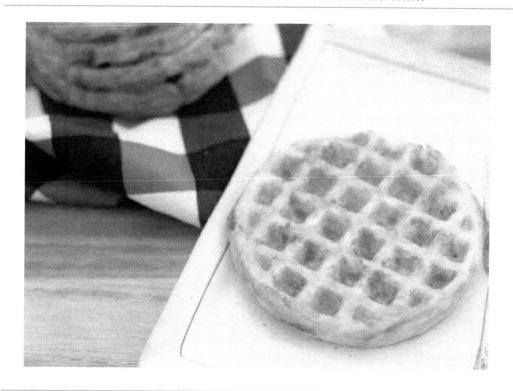

CARBS – **2 g** FAT – **13 g** PROTEIN – **10 g** CALORIES – **131**

Ingredients

- *1 large egg*
- *1 Tbsp blanched almond flour*
- *¼ tsp baking powder*
- *½ cup shredded mozzarella cheese*

Directions

1. Whisk egg, almond flour, and baking powder together.
2. Stir in mozzarella and set batter aside.
3. Turn on waffle maker to heat and oil it with cooking spray.
4. Pour half of the batter onto waffle maker and spread it evenly with a spoon.
5. Cook for 3 minutes, or until it reaches desired doneness.
6. Transfer to a plate and repeat with remaining batter.

7. Let chaffles cool for 2-3 minutes to crisp up.

OREO KETO CHAFFLES

SERVINGS: 2 PREP TIME: 5 min. COOK TIME: 5 min.

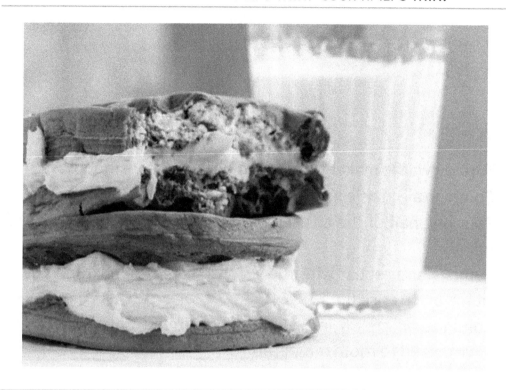

CARBS – 3 g FAT – 4 g PROTEIN – 7 g CALORIES – 66

Ingredients

- *1 egg*
- *1½ Tbsp unsweetened cocoa*
- *2 Tbsp lakanto monk fruit, or choice of sweetener*
- *1 Tbsp heavy cream*
- *1 tsp coconut flour*

½ tsp baking powder

½ tsp vanilla

FOR THE CHEESE CREAM:

- *1 Tbsp lakanto powdered sweetener*
- *2 Tbsp softened cream cheese*
- *¼ tsp vanilla*

Directions

1. Turn on waffle maker to heat and oil it with cooking spray.
2. Combine all chaffle ingredients in a small bowl.
3. Pour one half of the chaffle mixture into waffle maker. Cook for 3-5 minutes.
4. Remove and repeat with the second half if the mixture. Let chaffles sit for 2-3 to crisp up.
5. Combine all cream ingredients and spread on chaffle when they have cooled to room temperature.

GINGERBREAD CHAFFLE

SERVINGS: 2 PREP TIME: 5 min. COOK TIME: 5 min.

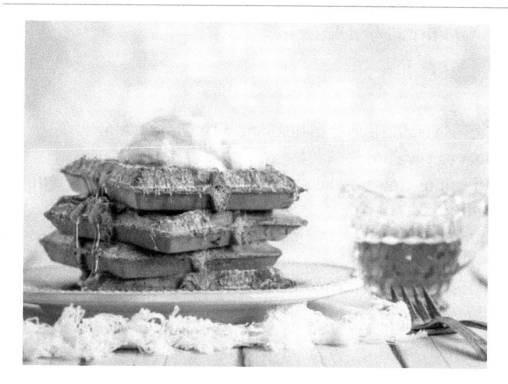

CARBS – 5 g FAT – 15 g PROTEIN – 12 g CALORIES – 103

Ingredients

- ½ cup mozzarella cheese grated
- 1 medium egg
- ½ tsp baking powder
- 1 tsp erythritol powdered
- ½ tsp ground ginger

¼ tsp ground nutmeg

½ tsp ground cinnamon

⅛ tsp ground cloves

2 Tbsp almond flour

- *1 cup heavy whipped cream ¼*
- *cup keto-friendly maple syrup*

Directions

1. Turn on waffle maker to heat and oil it with cooking spray.
2. Beat egg in a bowl.
3. Add flour, mozzarella, spices, baking powder, and erythritol. Mix well.
4. Spoon one half of the batter into waffle maker and spread out evenly.
5. Close and cook for 5 minutes.
6. Remove cooked chaffle and repeat with remaining batter.

-
-
-
-
-
-

7. Serve with whipped cream and maple syrup.

CHOCOLATE PEANUT BUTTER CHAFFLE

SERVINGS: 2 PREP TIME: 5 min. COOK TIME: 10 min.

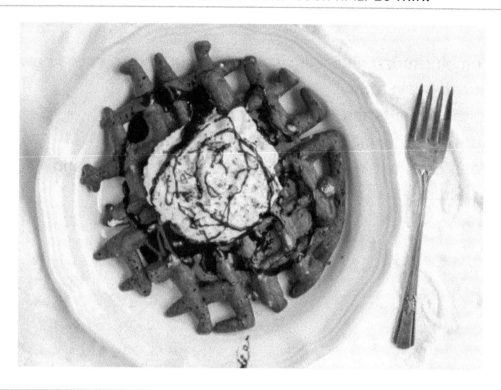

CARBS – 6 g FAT – 17 g PROTEIN – 15 g CALORIES – 236

Ingredients

- ½ cup shredded mozzarella cheese
- 1 Tbsp cocoa powder
- 2 Tbsp powdered sweetener
    2 Tbsp peanut butter
    ½ tsp vanilla

1 egg
2 Tbsp crushed peanuts
2 Tbsp whipped cream
¼ cup sugar-free chocolate syrup

Directions

1. Combine mozzarella, egg, vanilla, peanut butter, cocoa powder, and sweetener in a bowl.
2. Add in peanuts and mix well.
3. Turn on waffle maker and oil it with cooking spray.
4. Pour one half of the batter into waffle maker and cook for 4 minutes, then transfer to a plate.

-
-
-
-
-
-

5. Top with whipped cream, peanuts, and sugar-free chocolate syrup.

PUMPKIN PECAN CHAFFLES

SERVINGS: 2 PREP TIME: 10 min. COOK TIME: 10 min.

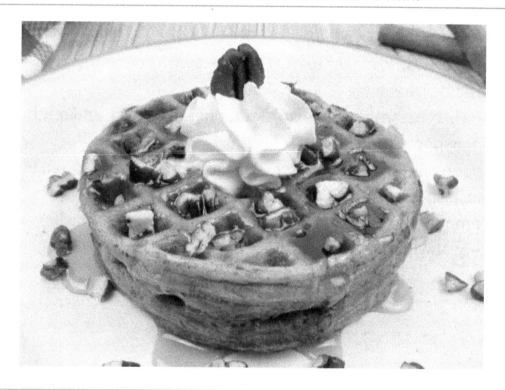

CARBS – 4 g FAT – 17 g PROTEIN – 11 g CALORIES – 210

Ingredients

- *1 egg*
- *½ cup mozzarella cheese grated*
- *1 Tbsp pumpkin puree*
   ½ tsp pumpkin spice
   1 tsp erythritol low carb sweetener

2 Tbsp almond flour
2 Tbsp pecans, toasted chopped
1 cup heavy whipped cream
¼ cup low carb caramel sauce

Directions

1. Turn on waffle maker to heat and oil it with cooking spray.
2. In a bowl, beat egg.
3. Mix in mozzarella, pumpkin, flour, pumpkin spice, and erythritol.
4. Stir in pecan pieces.
5. Spoon one half of the batter into waffle maker and spread evenly.
6. Close and cook for 5 minutes.
7. Remove cooked waffles to a plate.
8. Repeat with remaining batter.

9. Serve with pecans, whipped cream, and low carb caramel sauce.

ITALIAN CREAM CHAFFLE SANDWICH-CAKE

SERVINGS: 4 PREP TIME: 20 min. COOK TIME: 20 min.

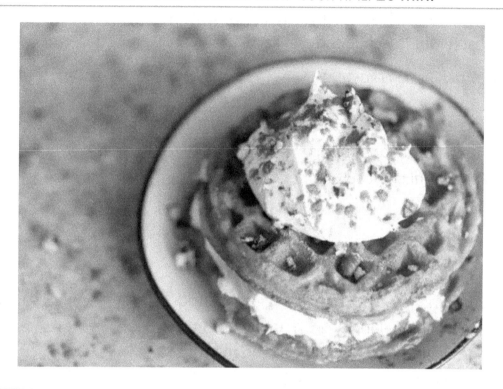

CARBS – 31 g FAT – 2 g PROTEIN – 5 g CALORIES – 168

Ingredients

- 4 oz cream cheese, softened, at room temperature
- 4 eggs
- 1 Tbsp melted butter
    1 tsp vanilla extract
    ½ tsp cinnamon

1 Tbsp monk fruit sweetener

4 Tbsp coconut flour

1 Tbsp almond flour

1½ teaspoons baking powder

- 1 Tbsp coconut, shredded and unsweetened
- 1 Tbsp walnuts, chopped

FOR THE ITALIAN CREAM FROSTING:

- 2oz cream cheese, softened, at room temperature
- 2 Tbsp butter room temp
- 2 Tbsp monk fruit sweetener
- ½ tsp vanilla

Directions

1. Combine cream cheese, eggs, melted butter, vanilla, sweetener, flours, and baking powder in a blender.
2. Add walnuts and coconut to the mixture.
3. Blend to get a creamy mixture.
4. Turn on waffle maker to heat and oil it with cooking spray.
5. Add enough batter to fill waffle maker. Cook for 2-3 minutes, until chaffles are done.
6. Remove and let them cool.
7. Mix all frosting ingredients in another bowl. Stir until smooth and creamy.
8. Frost the chaffles once they have cooled.
9. Top with cream and more nuts.

- # CHOCOLATE CHERRY CHAFFLES
-
-
-

SERVINGS: 1 PREP TIME: 5 min. COOK TIME: 5 min.

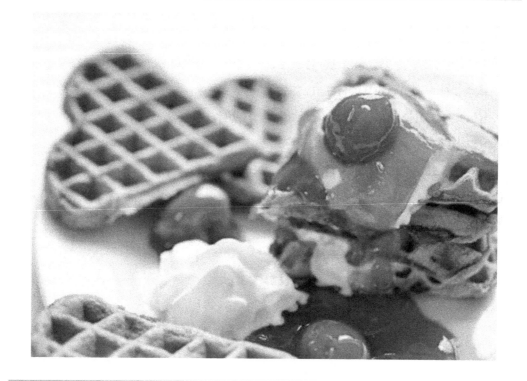

CARBS – 6 g FAT – 1 g PROTEIN – 1 g CALORIES – 130

Ingredients

- *1 Tbsp almond flour*
- *1 Tbsp cocoa powder*
- *1 Tbsp sugar free sweetener*
  - *½ tsp baking powder*
  - *1 whole egg*
  - *½ cup mozzarella cheese shredded*
  - *2 Tbsp heavy whipping cream whipped*

2 Tbsp sugar free cherry pie filling 1
Tbsp chocolate chips

Directions

1. Turn on waffle maker to heat and oil it with cooking spray.
2. Mix all dry components in a bowl.
3. Add egg and mix well.
4. Add cheese and stir again.
5. Spoon batter into waffle maker and close.
6. Cook for 5 minutes, until done.
7. Top with whipping cream, cherries, and chocolate chips.

BANANA NUT CHAFFLE

SERVINGS: 1 PREP TIME: 15 min. COOK TIME: 10 min.

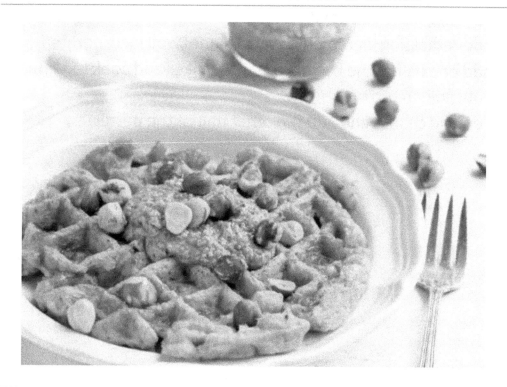

CARBS – 2 g FAT – 7 g PROTEIN – 8 g CALORIES – 119

Ingredients

- *1 egg*
- *1 Tbsp cream cheese, softened and room temp*
- *1 Tbsp sugar-free cheesecake pudding*
- *½ cup mozzarella cheese*
- *1 Tbsp monk fruit confectioners sweetener*

¼ tsp vanilla extract ¼
tsp banana extract
toppings of choice

Directions

1. Turn on waffle maker to heat and oil it with cooking spray.
2. Beat egg in a small bowl.
3. Add remaining ingredients and mix until well incorporated.
4. Add one half of the batter to waffle maker and cook for 4 minutes, until golden brown.
5. Remove chaffle and add the other half of the batter.

6. Top with your optional toppings and serve warm!

SAVORY CHAFFLES

BELGIUM CHAFFLES

SERVINGS: 1 PREP TIME: 5 min. COOK TIME: 6 min.

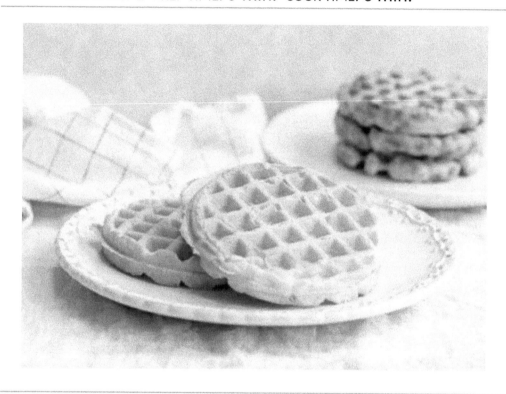

CARBS – 2 g FAT – 33 g PROTEIN – 44 g CALORIES – 460

Ingredients

- *2 eggs*
- *1 cup Reduced-fat Cheddar cheese, shredded*

Directions

1. Turn on waffle maker to heat and oil it with cooking spray.
2. Whisk eggs in a bowl, add cheese. Stir until well-combined.
3. Pour mixture into waffle maker and cook for 6 minutes until done.
4. Let it cool a little to crisp before serving.

BACON CHAFFLES

SERVINGS: 2 PREP TIME: 5 min. COOK TIME: 5 min.

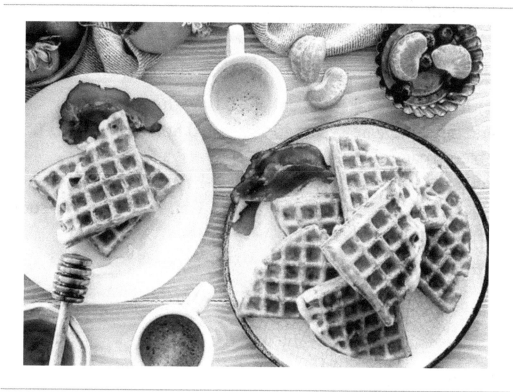

CARBS – 3 g FAT – 38 g PROTEIN – 23 g CALORIES – 446

Ingredients

- *2 eggs*
- *½ cup cheddar cheese*
- *½ cup mozzarella cheese*
- *¼ tsp baking powder ½*
- *Tbsp almond flour*
- *1 Tbsp butter, for waffle maker*

FOR THE FILLING:

- ¼ *cup bacon, chopped*
- *2 Tbsp green onions, chopped*

Directions

1. Turn on waffle maker to heat and oil it with cooking spray.
2. Add eggs, mozzarella, cheddar, almond flour, and baking powder to a blender and pulse 10 times, so cheese is still chunky.
3. Add bacon and green onions. Pulse 2-3 times to combine.
4. Add one half of the batter to the waffle maker and cook for 3 minutes, until golden brown.
5. Repeat with remaining batter.

6. Add your toppings and serve hot.

CRISPY BAGEL CHAFFLES

SERVINGS: 1 PREP TIME: 10 min. + day COOK TIME: 30 min.

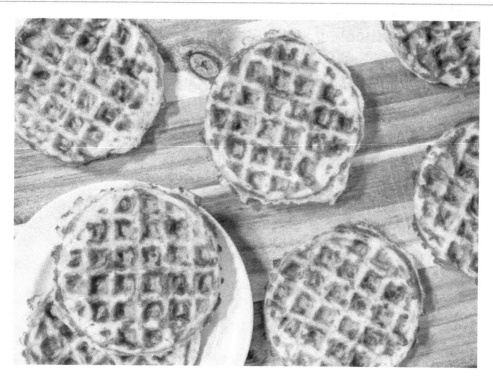

CARBS – 6 g FAT – 20 g PROTEIN – 21 g CALORIES – 287

Ingredients

- 2 eggs
- ½ cup parmesan cheese
- 1 tsp bagel seasoning
- ½ cup mozzarella cheese
- 2 teaspoons almond flour

Directions

1. Turn on waffle maker to heat and oil it with cooking spray.
2. Evenly sprinkle half of cheeses to a griddle and let them melt. Then toast for 30 seconds and leave them wait for batter.
3. Whisk eggs, other half of cheeses, almond flour, and bagel seasoning in a small bowl.
4. Pour batter into the waffle maker. Cook for 4 minutes.

5. Let cool for 2-3 minutes before serving.

BACON AND HAM CHAFFLE SANDWICH

SERVINGS: 2 PREP TIME: 10 min. COOK TIME: 5 min.

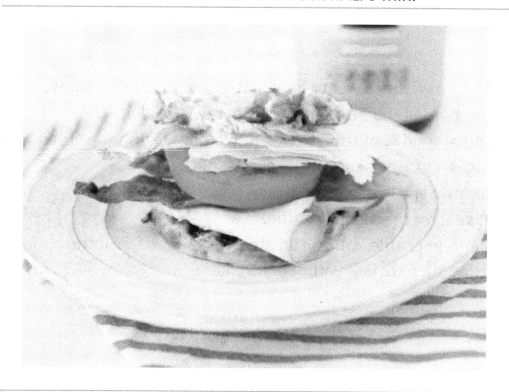

CARBS – 5 g FAT – 60 g PROTEIN – 31 g CALORIES – 631

Ingredients

- *3 egg*
- *½ cup grated Cheddar cheese*
- *1 Tbsp almond flour*
- *½ tsp baking powder*

FOR THE TOPPINGS:

- *4 strips cooked bacon*
- *2 pieces Bibb lettuce*
- *2 slices preferable ham*
- *2 slices tomato*

Directions

1. Turn on waffle maker to heat and oil it with cooking spray.
2. Combine all chaffle components in a small bowl.
3. Add around ¼ of total batter to waffle maker and spread to fill the edges. Close and cook for 4 minutes.
4. Remove and let it cool on a rack.
5. Repeat for the second chaffle.
6. Top one chaffle with a tomato slice, a piece of lettuce, and bacon strips, then cover it with second chaffle.

7. Plate and enjoy.

PARMESAN GARLIC CHAFFLE

SERVINGS: 2 PREP TIME: 5 min. COOK TIME: 5 min.

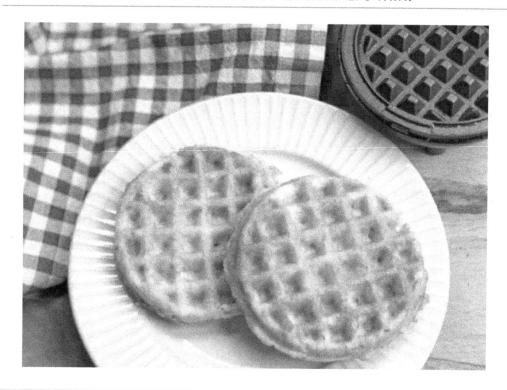

CARBS – 5 g FAT – 33 g PROTEIN – 19 g CALORIES – 385

Ingredients

- 1 Tbsp fresh garlic minced
- 2 Tbsp butter
- 1-oz cream cheese, cubed
- 2 Tbsp almond flour
- 1 tsp baking soda 2
- large eggs

1 tsp dried chives
½ cup parmesan cheese, shredded
¾ cup mozzarella cheese, shredded

Directions

1. Heat cream cheese and butter in a saucepan over medium-low until melted.
2. Add garlic and cook, stirring, for 2 minutes.
3. Turn on waffle maker to heat and oil it with cooking spray.
4. In a small mixing bowl, whisk together flour and baking soda, then set aside.
5. In a separate bowl, beat eggs for 1 minute 30 seconds on high, then add in cream cheese mixture and beat for 60 seconds more.
6. Add flour mixture, chives, and cheeses to the bowl and stir well.
7. Add ¼ cup batter to waffle maker.
8. Close and cook for 4 minutes, until golden brown.
9. Repeat for remaining batter.

10. Add favorite toppings and serve.

BUFFALO CHICKEN CHAFFLES

SERVINGS: 4 PREP TIME: 5 min. COOK TIME: 5 min.

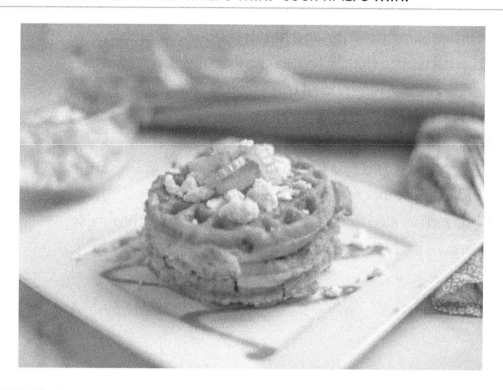

CARBS – 4 g FAT – 26 g PROTEIN – 22 g CALORIES – 337

Ingredients

- ¼ cup almond flour
- 1 tsp baking powder
- 2 large eggs
- ½ cup chicken, shredded
- ¾ cup sharp cheddar cheese, shredded
- ¼ cup mozzarella cheese, shredded
-
-

¼ cup Red-Hot Sauce + 1 Tbsp for topping
¼ cup feta cheese, crumbled
¼ cup celery, diced

Directions

1. Whisk baking powder and almond flour in a small bowl and set aside.
2. Turn on waffle maker to heat and oil it with cooking spray.
3. Beat eggs in a large bowl until frothy.
4. Add hot sauce and beat until combined.
5. Mix in flour mixture.
6. Add cheeses and mix until well combined.
7. Fold in chicken.
8. Pour batter into waffle maker and cook for 4 minutes.
9. Remove and repeat until all batter is used up.

10. Top with celery, feta, and hot sauce.

GARLIC CHEESE CHAFFLE BREAD STICKS

SERVINGS: 8 PREP TIME: 5 min. COOK TIME: 5 min.

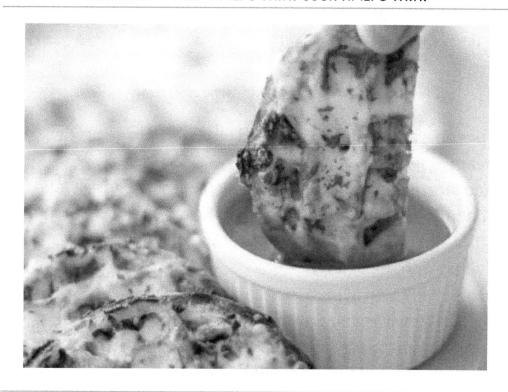

CARBS – 1 g FAT – 7 g PROTEIN – 4 g CALORIES – 74

Ingredients

- *1 medium egg*
- *½ cup mozzarella cheese, grated*
- *2 Tbsp almond flour*
- *½ tsp garlic powder*
- *½ tsp oregano*
- *½ tsp salt*

FOR THE TOPPINGS:

- *2 Tbsp butter, unsalted softened*
- *½ tsp garlic powder*
- *¼ cup grated mozzarella cheese 2*
- *tsp dried oregano for sprinkling*

Directions

1. Turn on waffle maker to heat and oil it with cooking spray.
2. Beat egg in a bowl.
3. Add mozzarella, garlic powder, flour, oregano, and salt, and mix.
4. Spoon half of the batter into the waffle maker.
5. Close and cook for 5 minutes. Remove cooked chaffle.
6. Repeat with remaining batter.
7. Place chaffles on a tray and preheat the grill.
8. Mix butter with garlic powder and spread over the chaffles.
9. Sprinkle mozzarella over top and cook under the broiler for 2-3 minutes, until cheese has melted.

CHAFFLE BRUSCHETTA

SERVINGS: 1 PREP TIME: 5 min. COOK TIME: 5 min.

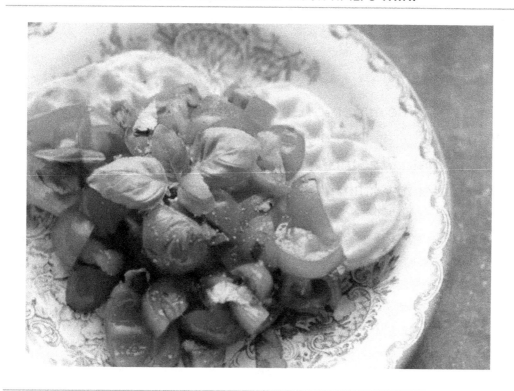

CARBS – 2 g FAT – 24 g PROTEIN – 34 g CALORIES – 352

Ingredients

- ½ cup shredded mozzarella cheese
- 1 whole egg beaten
- ¼ cup grated Parmesan cheese
- 1 tsp Italian Seasoning
- ¼ tsp garlic powder

FOR THE TOPPINGS:

- *3-4 cherry tomatoes, chopped*
- *1 tsp fresh basil, chopped*
- *Splash of olive oil Pinch*
- *of salt*

Directions

1. Turn on waffle maker to heat and oil it with cooking spray.
2. Whisk all chaffle ingredients, except mozzarella, in a bowl.
3. Add in cheese and mix.
4. Add batter to waffle maker and cook for 4-5 minutes.

5. Mix tomatoes, basil, olive oil, and salt. Serve over the top of chaffles.

PIZZA CHAFFLE

SERVINGS: 2 PREP TIME: 5 min. COOK TIME: 5 min.

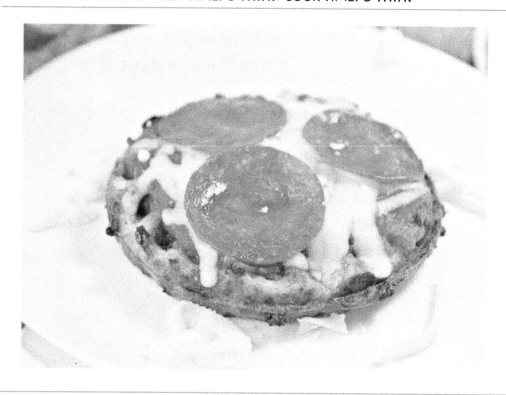

CARBS – 4 g FAT – 8g PROTEIN – 4 g CALORIES – 178

Ingredients

- *1 egg*
- *½ cup mozzarella cheese shredded*
- *Pinch of Italian seasoning 1 Tbsp no sugar*
- *added pizza sauce more shredded cheese,*
- *pepperoni for topping*

Directions

1. Turn on waffle maker to heat and oil it with cooking spray.
2. Mix egg and seasonings in a small bowl.
3. Mix in cheese.
4. Add 1 tsp cheese to hot waffle maker and melt for 30 seconds, then add half batter mixture to waffle maker and cook for 4 minutes, until golden brown.
5. Remove and repeat with remaining mixture.

6. Top with pizza sauce, cheese, and pepperoni. Microwave for 20 seconds on high and serve.

EGGS BENEDICT CHAFFLE

SERVINGS: 2 PREP TIME: 20 min. COOK TIME: 10 min.

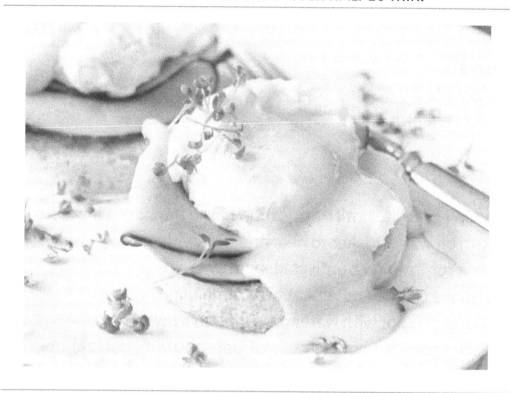

CARBS – 4 g FAT – 26 g PROTEIN – 26 g CALORIES – 365

Ingredients

FOR THE CHAFFLE:

- *2 egg whites*
- *2 Tbsp almond flour*
- *1 Tbsp sour cream*
- *½ cup mozzarella cheese*

FOR THE HOLLANDAISE:

- ½ cup salted butter
- 4 egg yolks
- 2 Tbsp lemon juice

FOR THE POACHED EGGS:

- 2 eggs
- 1 Tbsp white vinegar
- 3 oz deli ham

Directions

1. Whip egg white until frothy, then mix in remaining ingredients.
2. Turn on waffle maker to heat and oil it with cooking spray.
3. Cook for 7 minutes until golden brown.
4. Remove chaffle and repeat with remaining batter.
5. Fill half the pot with water and bring to a boil.
6. Place heat-safe bowl on top of pot, ensuring bottom doesn't touch the boiling water.
7. Heat butter to boiling in a microwave.
8. Add yolks to double boiler bowl and bring to boil.
9. Add hot butter to the bowl and whisk briskly. Cook until the egg yolk mixture has thickened.
10. Remove bowl from pot and add in lemon juice. Set aside.
11. Add more water to pot if needed to make the poached eggs (water should completely cover the eggs). Bring to a simmer. Add white vinegar to water.
12. Crack eggs into simmering water and cook for 1 minute 30 seconds. Remove using slotted spoon.

13. Warm chaffles in toaster for 2-3 minutes. Top with ham, poached eggs, and hollandaise sauce.

ZUCCHINI CHAFFLE

SERVINGS: 2 PREP TIME: 10 min. COOK TIME: 5 min.

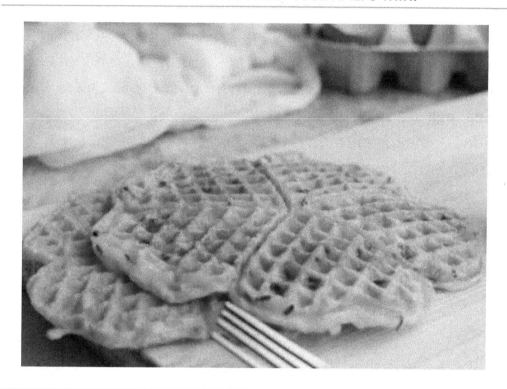

CARBS – 4 g FAT – 13 g PROTEIN – 16 g CALORIES – 194

Ingredients

- *1 cup grated zucchini*
- *1 egg*
- *½ cup shredded parmesan cheese*
- *¼ cup shredded mozzarella cheese*
-
-

¼ cup fresh basil, chopped ¾
tsp kosher salt, divided
½ tsp ground black pepper

Directions

1. Turn on waffle maker to heat and oil it with cooking spray.
2. Sprinkle ¼ tsp salt on zucchini, let it absorb for 2-3 minutes.
3. Wrap zucchini in a paper towel, then squeeze out excess water.
4. Beat egg in a small bowl.
5. Add zucchini, basil, mozzarella, ½ tsp salt, and pepper.
6. Sprinkle 1-2 Tbsp parmesan over the bottom of waffle maker.
7. Spread ¼ zucchini mixture on top of cheese. Top with 1-2 Tbsp parmesan and cook for 4-8 minutes, depending on waffle maker size.

8. Remove and repeat for remaining zucchini mixture.

BREAKFAST CHAFFLE

SERVINGS: 2 PREP TIME: 5 min. COOK TIME: 5 min.

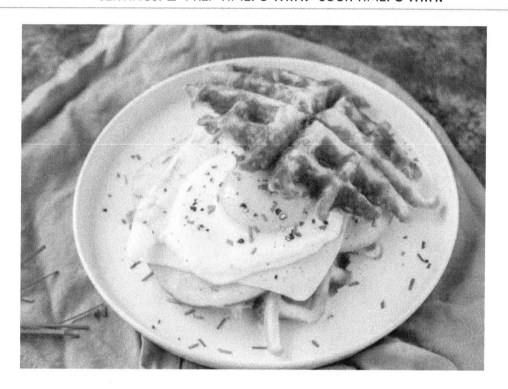

CARBS – 1 g FAT – 8 g PROTEIN – 9 g CALORIES – 115

Ingredients

- *2 eggs*
- *½ cup shredded mozzarella cheese*

FOR THE TOPPINGS:

- *2 ham slices*
- *1 fried egg*

Directions

1. Mix eggs and cheese in a small bowl.
2. Turn on waffle maker to heat and oil it with cooking spray.
3. Pour half of the batter into the waffle maker.
4. Cook for 2-4 minutes, remove, and repeat with remaining batter.
5. Place egg and ham between two chaffles to make a sandwich.

CHEDDAR JALAPEÑO CHAFFLE

SERVINGS: 2 PREP TIME: 5 min. COOK TIME: 5 min.

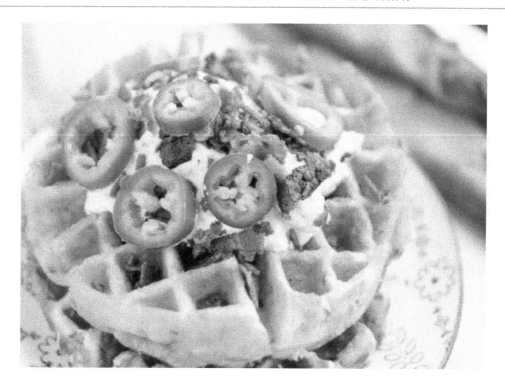

CARBS – 5 g FAT – 18 g PROTEIN – 18 g CALORIES – 307

Ingredients

- *2 large eggs*
- *½ cup shredded mozzarella*
- *¼ cup almond flour*
- *½ tsp baking powder*
- *¼ cup shredded cheddar cheese*

2 Tbsp diced jalapeños jarred or canned

FOR THE TOPPINGS:

- *½ cooked bacon, chopped*
- *2 Tbsp cream cheese*
- *¼ jalapeño slices*

Directions

1. Turn on waffle maker to heat and oil it with cooking spray.
2. Mix mozzarella, eggs, baking powder, almond flour, and garlic powder in a bowl.
3. Sprinkle 2 Tbsp cheddar cheese in a thin layer on waffle maker, and ½ jalapeño.
4. Ladle half of the egg mixture on top of the cheese and jalapeños.
5. Cook for 5 minutes, or until done.
6. Repeat for the second chaffle.

-
-
-

7. Top with cream cheese, bacon, and jalapeño slices.

BROCCOLI AND CHEESE CHAFFLES

SERVINGS: 1 PREP TIME: 5 min. COOK TIME: 5 min.

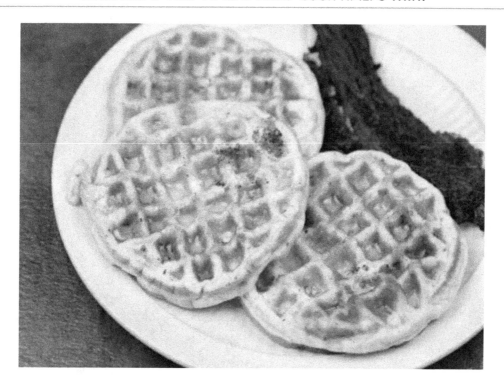

CARBS – 4 g FAT – 9 g PROTEIN – 7 g CALORIES – 125

Ingredients

- ⅓ cup raw broccoli, finely chopped
- ¼ cup shredded cheddar cheese
- 1 egg
    ½ tsp garlic powder
    ½ tsp dried minced onion
    Salt and pepper, to taste

Directions

1. Turn on waffle maker to heat and oil it with cooking spray.
2. Beat egg in a small bowl.
3. Fold in cheese, broccoli, onion, garlic powder, salt, and pepper.
4. Pour egg mixture into waffle maker. Cook for 4 minutes, or until done.
5. Remove from waffle maker with a fork.

6. Serve with sour cream or butter.

HASH BROWN CHAFFLE

SERVINGS: 2 PREP TIME: 20 min. COOK TIME: 10 min.

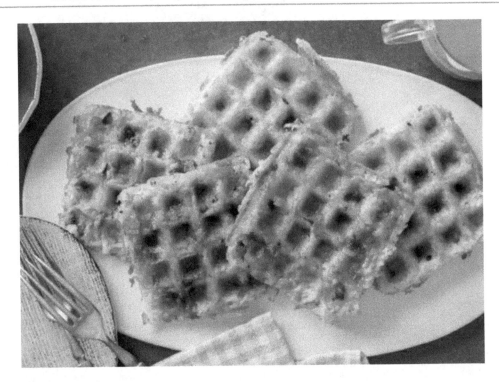

CARBS – 9 g FAT – 6 g PROTEIN – 4 g CALORIES – 194

Ingredients

- 1 large jicama root, *peeled and shredded*
- ½ medium onion, *minced*
- 2 garlic cloves, *pressed*

1.

   1 cup cheddar shredded cheese
   2 eggs
   Salt and pepper, to taste

Directions

Place jicama in a colander, sprinkle with 1-2 tsp salt, and let drain.
2. Squeeze out all excess liquid.
3. Microwave jicama for 5-8 minutes.
4. Mix ¾ of cheese and all other ingredients in a bowl.
5. Sprinkle 1-2 tsp cheese on waffle maker, add 3 Tbsp mixture, and top with 1-2 tsp cheese.
6. Cook for 5-6 minutes, or until done.
7. Remove and repeat for remaining batter.

8. Serve while hot with preferred toppings.

CHICKEN PARMESAN CHAFFLE

SERVINGS: 2 PREP TIME: 5 min. COOK TIME: 10 min.

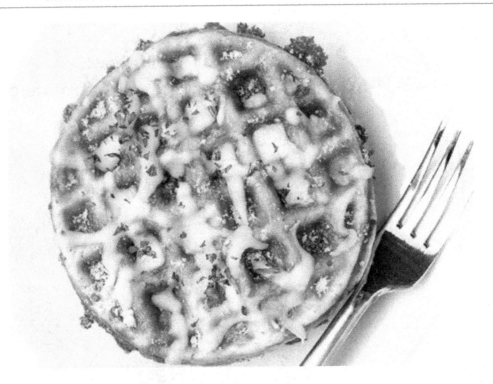

CARBS – 2g FAT – 13 g PROTEIN – 14 g CALORIES – 135

Ingredients

- ⅓ cup cooked chicken
- 1 egg
- ⅓ cup shredded mozzarella cheese

1.

¼ tsp basil, chopped
¼ garlic, minced
2 Tbsp tomato sauce
- *2 Tbsp mozzarella cheese*

Directions

Turn on waffle maker to heat and oil it with cooking spray.
2. Mix egg, basil, chicken, garlic, and ⅓ cup mozzarella in a small bowl.
3. Add half of the batter to the waffle maker and cook for 4 minutes, or until done.
4. Remove and repeat for remaining batter.
5. Let each chaffle sit for 2 minutes.
6. Top each chaffle with sauce and sprinkle with 2 Tbsp mozzarella cheese.
7. Preheat oven to 400°F and bake chaffles until cheese is melted.

TACO CHAFFLE SHELL

SERVINGS: 1 PREP TIME: 5 min. COOK TIME: 8 min.

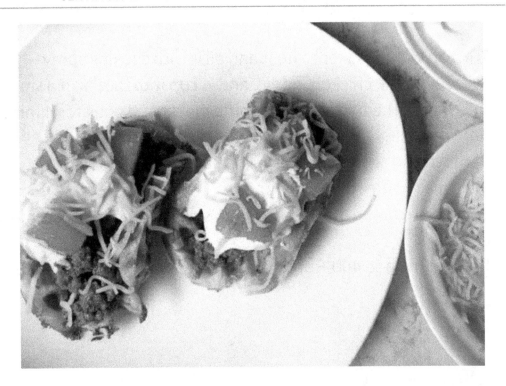

CARBS – 4 g FAT – 19 g PROTEIN – 18 g CALORIES – 258

Ingredients

- *1 egg white*
- *¼ cup shredded Monterey jack cheese*
- *¼ cup shredded sharp cheddar cheese*
- *¾ tsp water*
- *1 tsp coconut flour*

¼ tsp baking powder
⅛ tsp chili powder
Pinch of salt

Directions

1. Turn on waffle maker to heat and oil it with cooking spray.
2. Mix all components in a bowl.
3. Spoon half of the batter on the waffle maker and cook for 4 minutes.
4. Remove chaffle and set aside. Repeat for remaining chaffle batter.
5. Turn over a muffin pan and set chaffle between the cups to form a shell. Allow to set for 2-4 minutes.

6. Remove and serve with your favorite taco recipe.

PULLED PORK CHAFFLE

SERVINGS: **8** PREP TIME: **10 min.** COOK TIME: **8 h.**

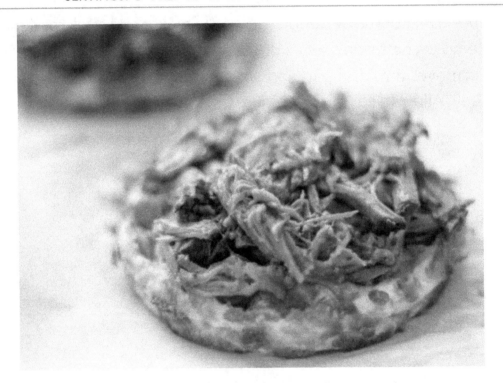

CARBS – **5 g** FAT – **14 g** PROTEIN – **36 g** CALORIES – **279**

Ingredients

- *1 cup shredded cheddar cheese*
- *2 eggs*
- *½ tsp BBQ Rub*
- *5 lbs pork butt*

¼ cup BBQ Rub

2 Tbsp yellow mustard

½ cup sweet BBQ Sauce

Directions

1. Brush mustard on each side of pork butt and season with rub.
2. Set smoker to 250°F. Smoke, uncovered, for about 4 hours, then wrap tightly, using butcher paper, and cook until internal temperature is 205°F.
3. Let pork rest for at least 1 hour before shredding it.
4. Mix cheese and eggs in a small bowl.
5. Scoop out ¼ cup of the mixture and pour into waffle maker. Cook for 5 minutes.

6. Top chaffles with shredded pork and BBQ sauce.

CHICKEN BACON CHAFFLE

SERVINGS: 2   PREP TIME: 5 min.   COOK TIME: 5 min.

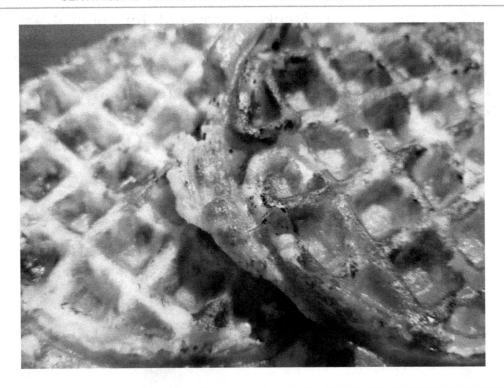

CARBS – 2 g   FAT – 14 g   PROTEIN – 16 g   CALORIES – 200

Ingredients

- 1 egg
- ⅓ cup cooked chicken, diced
- 1 piece of bacon, cooked and crumbled
- ⅓ cup shredded cheddar jack cheese

1 tsp powdered ranch dressing

Directions

1. Turn on waffle maker to heat and oil it with cooking spray.
2. Mix egg, dressing, and Monterey cheese in a small bowl.
3. Add bacon and chicken.
4. Add half of the batter to the waffle maker and cook for 3-4 minutes.
5. Remove and cook remaining batter to make a second chaffle.
6. Let chaffles sit for 2 minutes before serving.

CHAFFLE CUBAN SANDWICH

SERVINGS: 1 PREP TIME: 10 min. COOK TIME: 10 min.

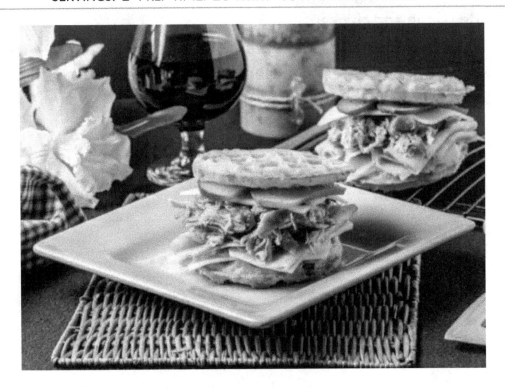

CARBS – 4 g FAT – 46 g PROTEIN – 33 g CALORIES – 522

Ingredients

- *1 large egg*
- *1 Tbsp almond flour*
- *1 Tbsp full-fat Greek yogurt*
- *⅛ tsp baking powder*
- *¼ cup shredded Swiss cheese*

FOR THE FILLING:

- *3 oz roast pork*
- *2 oz deli ham*
- *1 slice Swiss cheese*
- *3-5 sliced pickle chips*
- *½ Tbsp Dijon mustard*

Directions

1. Turn on waffle maker to heat and oil it with cooking spray.
2. Beat egg, yogurt, almond flour, and baking powder in a bowl.
3. Sprinkle ¼ Swiss cheese on hot waffle maker. Top with half of the egg mixture, then add ¼ of the cheese on top. Close and cook for 3-5 minutes, until golden brown and crispy.
4. Repeat with remaining batter.
5. Layer pork, ham, and cheese slice in a small microwaveable bowl. Microwave for 50 seconds, until cheese melts.

6. Spread the inside of chaffle with mustard and top with pickles. Invert bowl onto chaffle top so that cheese is touching pickles. Place bottom chaffle onto pork and serve.

SALMON CHAFFLES

SERVINGS: 2 PREP TIME: 10 min. COOK TIME: 10 min.

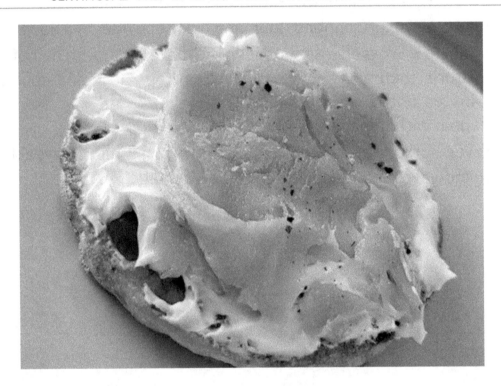

CARBS – 3 g FAT – 10 g PROTEIN – 5 g CALORIES – 201

Ingredients

- *1 large egg*
- *½ cup shredded mozzarella*
- *1 Tbsp cream cheese*
-
-

2 slices salmon

1 Tbsp everything bagel seasoning

Directions

1. Turn on waffle maker to heat and oil it with cooking spray.
2. Beat egg in a bowl, then add ½ cup mozzarella.
3. Pour half of the mixture into the waffle maker and cook for 3-4 minutes.
4. Remove and repeat with remaining mixture.

5. Let chaffles cool, then spread cream cheese, sprinkle with seasoning, and top with salmon.

CHAFFLE KATSU SANDWICH

SERVINGS: 4 PREP TIME: 30 min. + 2-4 days COOK TIME: 00 min.

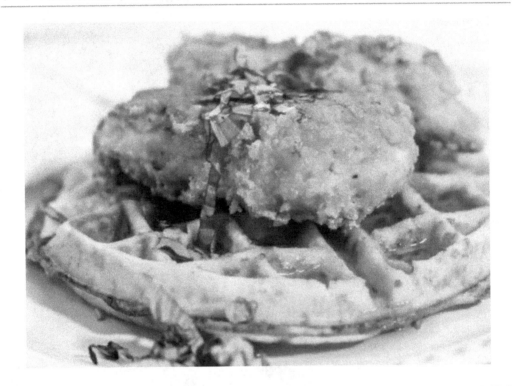

CARBS – 12 g FAT – 1 g PROTEIN – 2 g CALORIES – 57

Ingredients

FOR THE CHICKEN:

- ¼ lb boneless and skinless chicken thigh
- ⅛ tsp salt
- ⅛ tsp black pepper

½ cup almond flour

1 egg

3 oz unflavored pork rinds

2 cup vegetable oil for deep frying

FOR THE BRINE:

- 2 cup of water
- 1 Tbsp salt

FOR THE SAUCE:

- 2 Tbsp sugar-free ketchup
- 1½ Tbsp Worcestershire Sauce
- 1 Tbsp oyster sauce
- 1 tsp swerve/monkfruit

FOR THE CHAFFLE:

- 2 egg
- 1 cup shredded mozzarella cheese

Directions

1. Add brine ingredients in a large mixing bowl.
2. Add chicken and brine for 1 hour.
3. Pat chicken dry with a paper towel. Sprinkle with salt and pepper. Set aside.
4. Mix ketchup, oyster sauce, Worcestershire sauce, and swerve in a small mixing bowl.
5. Pulse pork rinds in a food processor, making fine crumbs.
6. Fill one bowl with flour, a second bowl with beaten eggs, and a third with crushed pork rinds.
7. Dip and coat each thigh in: flour, eggs, crushed pork rinds. Transfer on holding a plate.

8. Add oil to cover ½ inch of frying pan. Heat to 375°F.
9. Once oil is hot, reduce heat to medium and add chicken. Cooking time depends on the chicken thickness.
10. Transfer to a drying rack.
11. Turn on waffle maker to heat and oil it with cooking spray.
12. Beat egg in a small bowl.
13. Place ⅛ cup of cheese on waffle maker, then add¼ of the egg mixture and top with ⅛ cup of cheese.
14. Cook for 3-4 minutes.

15. Repeat for remaining batter.

16. Top chaffles with chicken katsu, 1 Tbsp sauce, and another piece of chaffle.

CAULIFLOWER CHAFFLE

SERVINGS: 3 PREP TIME: 5 min. COOK TIME: 1 min.

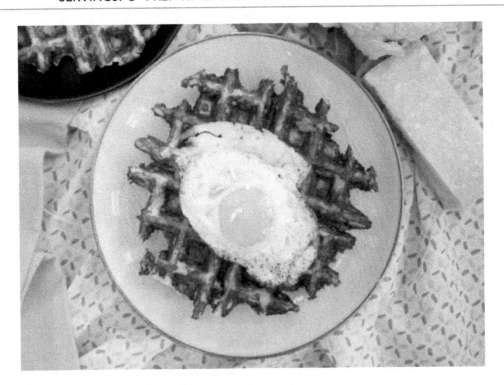

CARBS – 9 g FAT – 19 g PROTEIN – 22 g CALORIES – 304

Ingredients

- *2 cup cauliflower, minced*
- *2 cup shredded mozzarella cheese*
- *2 eggs*
- *2 Tbsp almond flour*
- *½ tsp paprika*

½ tsp onion powder
½ tsp oregano
Salt and pepper, to taste
3 egg for topping

Directions

1. Turn on waffle maker to heat and oil it with cooking spray.
2. Combine cauliflower, eggs, cheese, flour, onion powder, paprika, oregano, salt, and pepper.
3. Add 1 cup mixture to waffle maker. Cook for 6 minutes.
4. Remove the first chaffle, repeat with the remaining batter.
5. Fry eggs well.

6. Place a fried egg on top of each chaffle and serve.

VEGAN CHAFFLE

SERVINGS: **1** PREP TIME: **15 min.** COOK TIME: **25 min.**

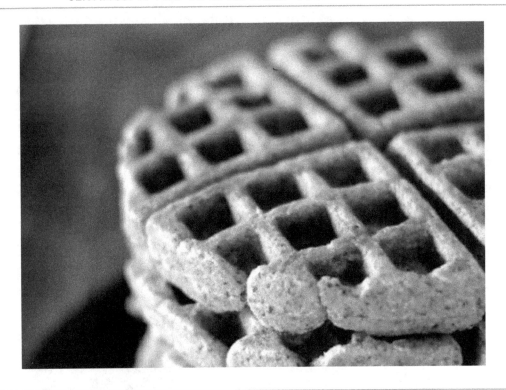

CARBS – **33 g** FAT – **25 g** PROTEIN – **25 g** CALORIES – **450**

Ingredients

- *1 Tbsp flaxseed meal*
- *2 ½ Tbsp water*
- *¼ cup low carb vegan cheese*
- *2 Tbsp coconut flour*
- *1 Tbsp low carb vegan cream cheese, softened Pinch of salt*

Directions

1. Turn on waffle maker to heat and oil it with cooking spray.
2. Mix flaxseed and water in a bowl. Leave for 5 minutes, until thickened and gooey.
3. Whisk remaining ingredients for chaffle.
4. Pour one half of the batter into the center of the waffle maker. Close and cook for 3-5 minutes.

5. Remove chaffle and serve.

TURKEY CHAFFLE SANDWICH

SERVINGS: 6 PREP TIME: 1 h. COOK TIME: 10 min.

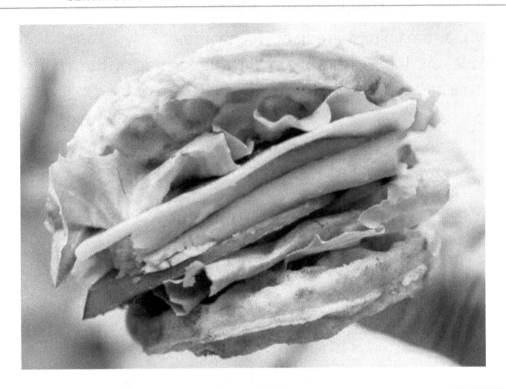

CARBS – 12 g FAT – 9 g PROTEIN – 11 g CALORIES – 246

Ingredients

- *2 egg whites*
- *2 Tbsp almond flour*
- *1 Tbsp mayonnaise*
- *1 tsp water*
- *¼ tsp baking powder Pinch of salt*

FOR THE SANDWICH:

- *2 Tbsp mayonnaise*
- *1 slice deli turkey*
- *1 slice cheddar cheese*
- *1 slice tomato*
- *1 leaf green leaf lettuce*

Directions

1. Turn on waffle maker to heat and oil it with cooking spray.
2. Mix all chaffle ingredients in a small bowl.
3. Pour half of the batter into waffle maker and cook for 3-5 minutes.
4. Remove and repeat with remaining batter.

5. Spread mayonnaise on one side of each chaffle. Layer on turkey, tomato and green leaf lettuce.

CHAFFLE BURGER

SERVINGS: 1 PREP TIME: 10 min. COOK TIME: 10 min.

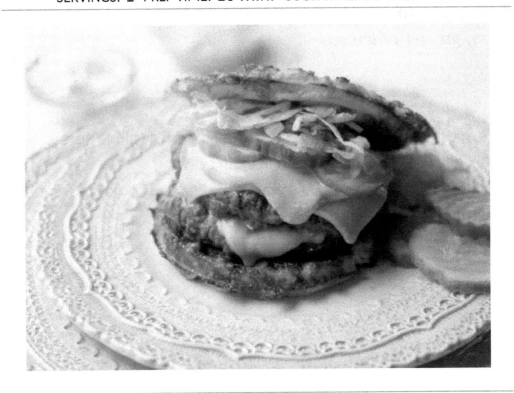

CARBS – 8 g FAT – 56 g PROTEIN – 65 g CALORIES – 831

Ingredients

FOR THE BURGER:

- *⅓ -pound ground beef*
- *½ tsp garlic salt*
- *2 slices American cheese*

FOR THE CHAFFLES:

- 1 large egg
- ½ cup shredded mozzarella
- ¼ tsp garlic salt

FOR THE SAUCE:

- 2 tsp mayonnaise
- 1 tsp ketchup1 tsp dill pickle relish
- splash vinegar, to taste

FOR THE TOPPINGS:

- 2 Tbsp shredded lettuce
- 3-4 dill pickles
- 2 tsp onion, minced

Directions

1. Heat a griddle over medium-high heat.
2. Divide ground beef into 2 balls and place on the griddle, 6 inches apart. Cook for 1 minute.
3. Use a small plate to flatten beef. Sprinkle with garlic salt.
4. Cook for 2-3, until halfway cooked through. Flip and sprinkle with garlic salt.
5. Cook for 2-3 minutes, or until cooked completely.
6. Place cheese slice over each patty and stack patties. Set aside on a plate. Cover with foil.
7. Turn on waffle maker to heat and oil it with cooking spray.
8. Whisk egg, cheese, and garlic salt until well combined.
9. Add half of the egg mixture to waffle maker and cook for 2-3 minutes.

10. Set aside and repeat with remaining batter.
11. Whisk all sauce ingredients in a bowl.
12. Top one chaffle with the stacked burger patties, shredded lettuce, pickles, and onions.
13. Spread sauce over the other chaffle and place sauce side down over the sandwich.
14. Eat immediately.

AIOLI CHICKEN CHAFFLE SANDWICH

SERVINGS: 1 PREP TIME: 10 min. COOK TIME: 6 min.

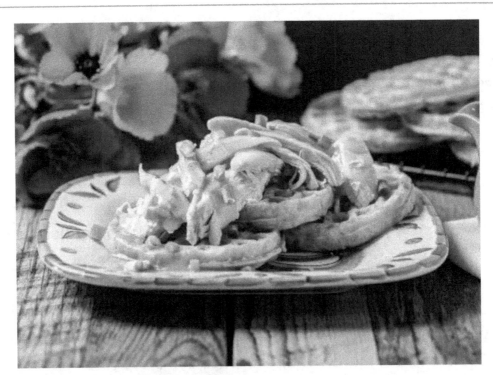

CARBS – 3 g FAT – 42 g PROTEIN – 34 g CALORIES – 545

Ingredients

- ¼ cup shredded rotisserie chicken
- 2 Tbsp Kewpie mayo ½
- tsp lemon juice
- 1 grated garlic clove
- ¼ green onion, chopped

  1 egg

  ½ cup shredded mozzarella cheese

Directions

1. Mix lemon juice and mayo in a small bowl.
2. Turn on waffle maker to heat and oil it with cooking spray.
3. Beat egg in a small bowl.
4. Place ⅛ cup of cheese on waffle maker, then spread half of the egg mixture over it and top with ⅛ cup of cheese. Close and cook for 3-4 minutes.
5. Repeat for remaining batter.

6. Place chicken on chaffles and top with sauce. Sprinkle with chopped green onion.

JAPANESE BREAKFAST CHAFFLE

SERVINGS: 2 PREP TIME: 5 min. COOK TIME: 10 min.

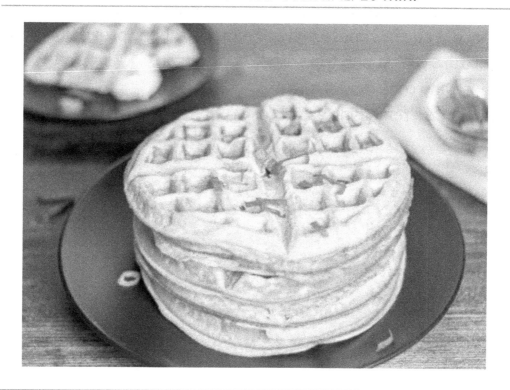

CARBS – 1 g FAT – 16 g PROTEIN – 8 g CALORIES – 183

Ingredients

- *1 egg*
- *½ cup shredded mozzarella cheese*

1 Tbsp kewpie mayo
1 stalk of green onion, chopped
1 slice bacon, chopped

Directions

1. Turn on waffle maker to heat and oil it with cooking spray. 2 Beat egg in a small bowl.
3. Add 1 Tbsp mayo, bacon, and ½ green onion. Mix well.
4. Place ⅛ cup of cheese on waffle maker, then spread half of the egg mixture over it and top with ⅛ cup cheese.
5. Close and cook for 3-4 minutes.
6. Repeat for remaining batter.

7. Transfer to a plate and sprinkle with remaining green onion.

SCALLION CREAM CHEESE CHAFFLE

SERVINGS: 2 PREP TIME: 15 min. + 1 h. COOK TIME: 20 min.

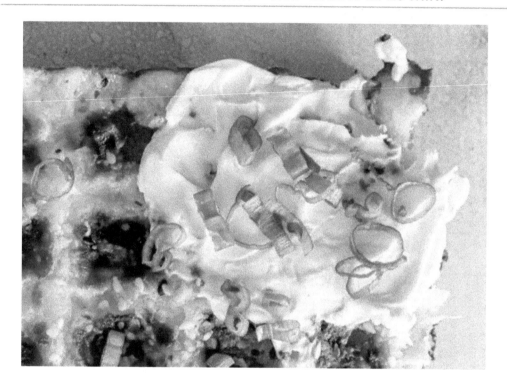

CARBS – 8 g FAT – 11 g PROTEIN – 5 g CALORIES – 168

Ingredients

- *1 large egg*
- *½ cup of shredded mozzarella*
- *2 Tbsp cream cheese*

1 Tbsp everything bagel seasoning
1-2 sliced scallions

Directions

1. Turn on waffle maker to heat and oil it with cooking spray.
2. Beat egg in a small bowl.
3. Add in ½ cup mozzarella.
4. Pour half of the mixture into the waffle maker and cook for 3-4 minutes.
5. Remove chaffle and repeat with remaining mixture.

6. Let them cool, then cover each chaffle with cream cheese, sprinkle with seasoning and scallions.

GRILLED CHEESE CHAFFLE

SERVINGS: 1 PREP TIME: 10 min. COOK TIME: 10 min.

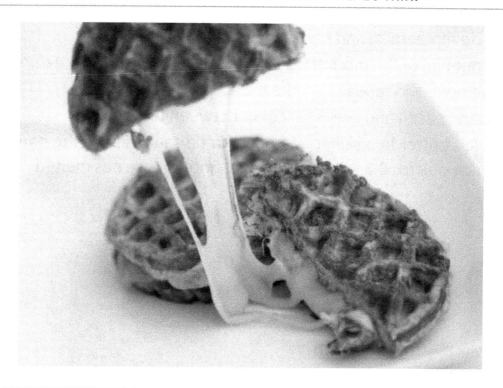

CARBS – 4 g FAT – 18 g PROTEIN – 7 g CALORIES – 233

Ingredients

- *1 large egg*
- *½ cup mozzarella cheese*
-
-
-
-

2 slices yellow American cheese
2-3 slices cooked bacon, cut in half
1 tsp butter
½ tsp baking powder

Directions

1. Turn on waffle maker to heat and oil it with cooking spray.
2. Beat egg in a bowl.
3. Add mozzarella, and baking powder.
4. Pour half of the mix into the waffle maker and cook for 4 minutes.
5. Remove and repeat to make the second chaffle.
6. Layer bacon and cheese slices in between two chaffles.
7. Melt butter in a skillet and add chaffle sandwich to the pan. Fry on each side for 2-3 minutes covered, until cheese has melted.

8. Slice in half on a plate and serve.

AVOCADO CHAFFLE

SERVINGS: 2   PREP TIME: 10 min.   COOK TIME: 10 min.

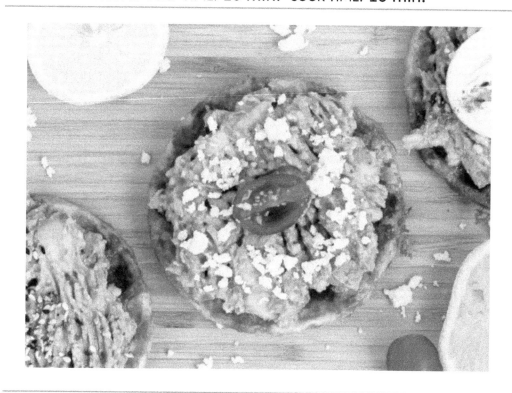

CARBS – 5 g   FAT – 19 g   PROTEIN – 7 g   CALORIES – 232

Ingredients

- ½ avocado, sliced
- ½ tsp lemon juice
- ⅛ tsp salt

⅛ tsp black pepper
1 egg
½ cup shredded cheese
¼ crumbled feta cheese
1 cherry tomato, halved

Directions

1. Mash together avocado, lemon juice, salt, and pepper until wellcombined.
2. Turn on waffle maker to heat and oil it with cooking spray.
3. Beat egg in a small mixing bowl.
4. Place ⅛ cup of cheese on waffle maker, then spread half of the egg mixture over it and top with ⅛ cup of cheese.
5. Close and cook for 3-4 minutes. Repeat for remaining batter.
6. Let chaffles cool for 3-4 minutes, then spread avocado mix on top of each.

7. Top with crumbled feta and cherry tomato halves.

CONCLUSION

Thank you for reading this book and having the patience to try the recipes.

I do hope that you have had as much enjoyment reading and experimenting with the meals as I have had writing the book.